Sugar and Obesity:

is *fructose* the culprit?

G. C. Cook

MD, DSc, FRCP, FRCPE, FRACP, FLS

Visiting Professor, University College London

Annie

With Best Wishes

Gordon Cook

19 : vi : 2018.

Published by

MELROSE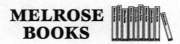
BOOKS

An Imprint of Melrose Press Limited
St Thomas Place, Ely
Cambridgeshire
CB7 4GG, UK
www.melrosebooks.co.uk

FIRST EDITION

Copyright © G C Cook 2017

The Author asserts his moral right to
be identified as the author of this work

Cover designed by Melrose Books

ISBN **978-1-912026-91-3 hardback**
        978-1-912026-92-0 epub
        978-1-912026-93-7 mobi

Printed and bound in Great Britain by:
4edge Limited
22 Eldon Way, Eldon Way Industrial Estate
Hockley, Essex
SS5 4AD

This book is dedicated to the memory of the late John Yudkin (1910–95), who rightly pointed out the huge recent increase in '*refined-sugar*' consumption by *Homo sapiens*, and its probable consequences for human disease.

The whole world is in the grip of an *obesity pandemic*. While the bulk of evidence invokes '*refined-sugar*' as the principal culprit, it is important to keep an open mind concerning alternative possibilities. As a *Times* columnist has indicated, items historically in common usage, accepted in their day as risk-free, have since proved this *not* to be the case. Two commodities which the writer had in mind were lead in Queen Elizabeth I (1533–1603)'s beauty products, and cigarettes prescribed for a 'weak chest' – both of which are now known to be carcinogenic. [H Rumbelow. Could things we do every day give us cancer? *Times 2, Lond* 2015; September 7: 6–7.]

Books by the same author:

Acute Renal Failure *ed* (1964)

Tropical Gastroenterology (1980)

100 Clinical Problems in Tropical Medicine (1987)

Communicable and Tropical Disease (1988)

Parasitic Disease in Clinical Practice (1990)

From the Greenwich Hulks to Old St Pancras: a history of tropical disease in London (1992) (reissued 2015)

Gastroenterological Problems from the Tropics (1995)

Travel-associated Disease (1995)

Manson's Tropical Diseases – 20th *ed* (1996)

100 Clinical Problems in Tropical Medicine – 2nd *ed* (1998)

Manson's Tropical Diseases – 21st *ed* (2003)

Victorian Incurables: a history of the Royal Hospital for Neuro-disability, Putney (2004)

John MacAlister's Other Vision: a history of the Fellowship of Postgraduate Medicine (2005)

The Incurables Movement: an illustrated history of the British Home (2006)

Tropical Medicine: an illustrated history of the pioneers (2007)

Disease in the Merchant Navy: a history of the Seamen's Hospital Society (2007)

Health-care for All: history of a third-world dilemma (2009)

Caribbean Disease: Dr George Low's expedition in 1901–02 (2009)

Manson's Tropical Diseases – 22nd *ed* (2009)

Twenty-six Portland Place: the early years of the Royal Society of Tropical Medicine and Hygiene (2011)

Torrid Disease: memoirs of a tropical physician in the late twentieth century (2011)

Origin of a Medical Specialty: the Seamen's Hospital Society and tropical medicine (2012)

The Tropical Disease that never existed: a history of sprue (2013)

The Rise and Fall of a Medical Specialty: London's clinical tropical medicine (2014)

National Service Fifty Years Ago: life of a medical conscript in West Africa (2014)

Disease and Sanitation in Victorian Britain: lessons for the 'Third World' (2015)

Before the 'Germ Theory': a history of cause and management of infectious disease before 1900 (2015)

The Milk Enzyme: adventures with the human *lactase* polymorphism (2016)

History of malabsorption in a warm environment (2016)

Greenwich and its lost hospitals: havens of maritime welfare (2017)

[Headings in bold font indicate titles published by Melrose Books]

CONTENTS

PREFACE

The world is currently in the grip of an obesity *pandemic*. Being fat is now considered by many to be the *normal* state for Britain's population. Although '*refined-sugar*', coupled with a steep reduction in physical activity is favoured by most as the likely cause, that opinion is by no means unanimous and the *sugar industry* in this respect refuses to lie low. This book highlights the crisis, its cause(s) and also reflects on possible solutions.

When I was a child (in the 1930s), being overweight, or obese, was regarded by many as a sign of healthiness, wisdom being that tuberculosis ('phthisis') was so common in Britain that an indication of fitness was being overweight; also, obesity was frequently categorised as a 'glandular disorder' even though other evidence of Cushing's syndrome or any other endocrine abnormality was, for example, lacking! Obesity is now considered one of the most common (if not the commonest) and important diseases in the world.[1]

It is *not* now however, confined to affluent sections of a population as in the past, but poor and underprivileged people are also involved;[2] urgent action must therefore be taken. One estimate is that *obesity* and its complications costs the British *National Health Service* (NHS) £5 billion annually, a figure which has *not* so far been significantly diminished by *public health* campaigns; so vast is this problem that the very future of the NHS itself is at stake.[3]

Obesity is defined by the *Shorter Oxford English Dictionary* (OED) as:

> The condition of being obese; corpulence (1610 Fr *obesité* or L. obesitas, f *obesus*),

and **Obese** as:

> Very fat or fleshy, corpulent (-L *obesus*, that has eaten himself fat, stout, plump …).

ix

Until recently, being overweight or, in exceptional cases, *morbidly* obese (*see* Prologue), was relatively unusual in the 'developing' or 'third world' – in part as a result of widespread presence of *malnutrition* and *infectious disease*; in contrast, being overweight or obese is presently commonplace universally.

An article in the London *Times* newspaper in May 2014 was extremely alarming: '*75% of British men will be obese by 2030*'; two thirds of women [it continued], will also fall into this category, while at present 66% of British men and 57% of women are *already* either overweight or obese'. Ireland was likely to become Europe's 'fattest nation' it claimed, while the Czech Republic, Poland, Spain and the UK [are] not far behind'. This article was apparently based on a 'Europe-wide study', also involving the *World Health Organisation* (WHO); the bulk of evidence for the crisis being largely 'blamed on the government's *laissez-faire* approach to regulating food sales.'[4] Another contribution titled: 'UK is a nation of fatties …' was accompanied by a leading article: 'Eat less …'. This obesity pandemic is … in fact currently raging throughout the UK and indeed the whole world.[5]

Two major alterations in lifestyle within *Homo sapiens* have emerged in recent decades: an alteration in eating habits, and a significant decline in exercise. Under the former heading should be noted, an enormous increase in '*refined-sugar*' (sucrose) consumption. It is important to stress that in this context, '*refined-sugar*' indicates *sucrose* and *not* another saccharide.[6]

But is '*refined-sugar* in fact the major cause? As this book will attempt to establish, this is by far the most likely nutritional component to be involved, although not all agree. Several theories exist as to why sucrose *causes* obesity. There are, for example, some based upon appetite hormones (*see* Chapter 9), and others implicating colonic bacteria (*see* Chapter 4). Most are based on the simple premise that *total* calories are responsible. The author of this book is of the opinion that because the two moieties of sucrose are handled independently and differently, it is an excess of the *fructose* component (*see* Chapter 8) which is the ultimate dietary trigger of obesity, rather than *total* calories. The glucose moiety after all is essential for life in *all* mammalia, and is clearly devoid of serious side-effects. All fruits of course contain *fructose*, but at a relatively low concentration compared with the colossal concentration in 'refined-sugar'; as for honey, its major sweetener is also fructose, but that is consumed in an entirely different manner to that of 'refined-sugar' compounds (see Chapter 5). Thus, fructose is both metabolised in the human body differently from glucose (see Chapter 8), and furthermore its concentration in the diet of H sapiens (particularly in childhood) has escalated in recent years.[7]

Following discovery of hormones associated with appetite – leptin and ghrelin – in the 1990s (see Chapter 9), a great deal of emphasis moved away from simple dietary items (ie, carbohydrates, and formerly also fats) to physiological factors as major underlying causes of obesity. Colonic bacteria have also come to the fore in recent research, a possibility which will be discussed in Chapter 4. Abnormalities within the body, rather than food constituents themselves, the theories claim, precede obesity. This book seeks to throw the discussion back to dietary components, headed by a huge intake of sucrose which at high concentration has historically been alien in evolution of all mammals – fructose. Increasing concentration of 'refined-sugar' in most present-day diets has been highlighted in Times reports.[8] John Yudkin in a 1960s 'best-selling' book in which many, but by no means all, arguments are sound, concentrated predominantly on an association between a high 'refined-sugar' intake and arterial disease, with excessive weight and obesity lower down his list of undesirable consequences. Most discussion related to total calories and vital nutrients including numerous 'toxic' effects of excessive sucrose. Despite these provisos, Yudkin powerfully stressed the ill-effects of an excess of 'refined-sugar' in human diets.[9]

Why though, did H sapiens in relatively recent times turn to ingestion of 'refined-sugar' in these huge amounts? Matt Ridley (as well as others) provide a plausible answer. Ancel Keys (1904–2004) (see Chapter 12), an American 'scientist' managed to 'hoodwink' the medical establishment the world over into believing that a fatty diet was the major exogenous cause of coronary artery disease, and later that dietary cholesterol, was instrumental in its pathogenesis. Keys' work suggesting that dietary fat and cholesterol were both implicated in production of atherosclerosis, is now acknowledged to have been both fraudulent and dishonest. Ingestion of 'refined-sugar' as an alternative calorie source was the result, and this is possibly a major reason why the world is currently facing this huge *obesity epidemic*.[10]

Also, not only is the British public discarding twice as much food overall as is the case with several other European countries, but nearly fifty per cent of *fruit and vegetables*, and *not* sugary items, is being wasted, according to an article in *Environmental Research Letters*.[11]

It is also pertinent to stress again the *cost* to Britain (*eg*, £4.2 billion in 2007) of the epidemic. The Chief Executive of Britain's NHS has recently indicated that obesity and its complications were costing more than the Police and Fire services of Britain put together. A proposed tax on 'sugary drinks' (*see* Chapter 15) will help tackle this issue in a way similar to reduction in salt intake – which reduced NHS costs by about £1.5 billion over 15 years.[12]

In this book therefore, my intention has been to demonstrate that lifestyle changes which have recently affected daily living, including lack of exercise, is introduction of sudden and monumental peaks of blood-*fructose* – derived from 'fast' food and 'fizzy' drinks and *not* merely *total calories* – entering the circulation. It is likely that modern *H sapiens* cannot cope with these vast amounts of *fructose* which have accounted for both a sudden increase in obesity, and escalating levels of *gout* (*see* Chapter 11 and Epilogue). It is this, in my opinion, as well as inactivity, which is the major causative factor in weight-gain and obesity in the majority of individuals. Newer theories incorporating hormones and colonic bacteria probably have only minor relevance, the major culprit undoubtedly being *fructose*. It seems most unlikely that this 'foreign' carbohydrate (*refined-sugar*)will be abandoned[13] however, and the NHS will continue to take the strain![14]

There is a minority who still considers that being obese is a good thing, while others consider it a significant factor in limitation of longevity; both views will be addressed in this book.[15]

I again thank Maureen Moran for her skilful typing, and Gwyneth Law of Melrose Books for correction of numerous errors in my final typescript.

G C Cook.
St Albans, May 2017

References and notes

1   C Smyth. Now it's normal to be fat, warns Britain's health chief. *Times, Lond* 2014; March 28: 3; K Lay. Obesity as dangerous as terror threat, warns medical chief. *Ibid* 2015; December 11: 2; K Lay. Britons are sugar addicts, says minister. *Ibid* 2017; February 8: 12. (*See also*: H Rumbelow. A fat, weighty debate about your life. *Times 2, Lond* 2016; May 12: 2–3.)

2   S Baxter. Obesity isn't an act of terrorism, it's a product of affluence. *Sunday Times, Lond* 2015; December 13: 26. (*See also*: Anonymous. Obesity link to poverty. *Times, Lond* 2017; January 11: 4; C Smyth. Obesity spreads to world's poorest. *Ibid* 2014; January 3: 9.)

3   Anonymous. Obesity's huge cost. *Ibid* 2016; June 8; 4; C Smyth. Obesity crisis could ruin us, NHS boss says. *Ibid* 2015: May 19: 17.

4   O Moody. 75% of British men "will be obese by 2030". *Ibid* 2014; May 10: 4.

5   N Woolcock. UK is a nation of fatties at risk from infectious disease. *Ibid* 2015: April 9: 4; Anonymous. Eat less: Britain is a fine place to live but its population needs to stop the growth of obesity. *Ibid* 2015: April 9: 27.

6   Anonymous. Sweet and sour: sugar has joined the long list of things that are bad for us. *Ibid* 2014; January 25: 22; E Roberts. Sugar rush. *Ibid* 2014; January 28: 29.

7   G C Cook. Absorption and metabolism of D(-) fructose in man. *Am J clin Nut* 1971: 24; 1302–7; G Taubes. The science of obesity: what do we really know about what makes us fat? *Br med J* 2013 April 20; 346: 16–19; G Taubes. *The case against sugar.* London; Portobello Books 2016: 365; G Jones. Sugar. *Times, Lond* 2014; January 14: 27; A Boyd. Don't blame sugar. *Ibid* 2015; September 7: 32; Correspondence. Challenging conventional wisdom on obesity. *Ibid* 2016; May 28: 28.

8   C Smyth. Dump the lumps with sugar swaps, urge health chiefs. *Ibid* 2015; January 5: 4.

9   J Yudkin. *Pure, white and deadly: how sugar is killing us and what we can do to stop it.* London: Penguin Books 1986: 200; M McCarthy. High sugar intake is linked to raised risk of cardiovascular mortality. *Br med J* 2014; 348: 5.

10 N Teicholz. *The Big Fat Surprise: why butter, meat, and cheese belong to a healthy diet.* London: Scribe Publications 2015: 369; M Ridley. More eggs, please. Cholesterol is OK now: this u-turn on dietary advice is long overdue. All kinds of damage have been done to people's lives and livelihoods. *Times, Lond* 2015; May 25: 23.

11 B Webster. Wasteful Britons bin nearly half of fruit and vegetables. *Ibid* 2015; August 12: 4. K Burgess. À la carte falls off the menus as chefs cut food waste. *Ibid* 2016; January 21: 11; T Stuart. Supermarkets must raise their game to stop food waste. *Ibid* 2017; March 9: 26; C Smyth. Cancer patients 'will suffer in NHS war on waste'. *Ibid* 2017; March 29: 12. (*See also*: Anonymous. Waste Not: we are morally diminished by our wastefulness of food. *Ibid* 2015; August 12: 27; O Moody. Spies in your fridge will show how much food is thrown away. *Ibid* 2015; November 12: 25; G Keate. Pledge to cut food waste will provide 60m meals for poor. *Ibid* 2017; January 24: 2.)

12 B Green. Burn off the sugar. *Ibid* 2014; June 30: 29.

13 J Turner. We are too sweet on sugar to give it up easily: the way to kick the habit is to cut down on the stuff hidden in pasta sauce, ready meals and fizzy drinks. *Ibid* 2014; January 11: 23;

14 Op cit. *See* note 3 (anonymous) above.

15 M Bateson. Being overweight is 'good for health'. *Ibid* 2017; March 10: 3.

PROLOGUE

Obesity is usually a *preventable* disease in which there is an excessive fat accumulation in all parts of the body imposing a potentially negative effect on health; that applies not only to *Homo sapiens* but to *all* mammalia. Individuals are by definition categorised as *obese* when the body mass index (BMI) – *ie,* body weight divided by the square of his/her height – exceeds 30 kg m^2. Although a figure of 20–25 is associated with the lowest mortality rate, one greater than 32 predicts a doubled one. A figure of >40 might be an indication for bariatric surgery (*see* Chapter 15)[1] and reduces life-expectancy by an average of *ten* years. There are now more individuals worldwide with a BMI of >30 than those who are under-nourished![2]

Historically, the disease was recognised by Hippocrates (c 470–400 BC), and later considered by the ancient Indian physician Sushruta Samhita in the *sixth* century BC to be related to heart disease and *type-2-diabetes mellitus*. Numerous cases of obesity have since occurred historically, but arguably one of the most documented examples is King Henry VIII (1491–1547) who suffered from gluttony (the *seventh* deadly sin) in mature years having earlier suffered a hypothalamic lesion – whilst taking part in a jousting contest[3] – which probably caused this anomaly. For most of history however, mankind has struggled with food *scarcity*, and obesity was not therefore a major problem, except in certain individuals – most in more affluent sections of society. During the *nineteenth* century, weight (as well as height) of military and other personnel assumed higher dimensions than hitherto, and a rise in obesity was predicted; numerous cases of obesity were later recorded in the *twentieth* century and beyond. In recent times, it is clear that it was 'high quality' newspapers which were first to recognise pre-obesity.[4] So common in fact has the condition become that many regard obesity as the *norm*, while numerous others are 'in denial'. One practical problem in management is that general practitioners are frequently reluctant to address this problem with their patients.[5]

Obesity is ultimately caused by an imbalance between input (calories) and output (*ie,* usually lack of physical activity – *see* Chapter 4), but genetic predisposition, and endocrine/psychiatric factors occasionally enter the equation. Using the mid-*nineteenth* century English phrase: '*An apple a day keeps the doctor away*', the technology firm with that name has recently launched an *app* designed to monitor both weight-gain and degree of exercise.[6] Insufficient sleep has been incriminated (*see* Chapters 4 and 9), as has greater time spent in viewing either television or videos (especially in children); less time designated to playing games and sports in schools has undoubtedly contributed.

Obesity in the past

H sapiens has throughout recorded history sought a sweetener in his/ her food (*see* Chapter 5). Thus in the days of honey (*ie,* before wide-spread introduction of '*refined-sugar*' [sucrose] into the human diet – *see* Chapter 6) a total of 21 entries in the *Oxford Dictionary of Quotations* are relevant to this naturally occurring substance – five in the Bible, and another five in the writings of William Shakespeare (1564–1616) – while a mere four refer to *sugar* (two of which also possess a Shakespearian origin).[7] As this book will indicate, '*refined-sugar*' – derived from either sugar cane or -beet – gradually succeeded honey and presently constitutes a major dietary item. For those seeking an alternative, a miscellany of synthetic sweeteners (*see* Chapter 14) – many associated with significant side-effects – has reached the market-place.

In historical recording, average *height* has received far more attention than *weight*. In an assessment of British men – the height of whom correlates closely with childhood nutrition – over the last 1,000 years, average height has been fairly constant at 5ft 8in (173 cm) – 5ft 10in (176 cm), apart from significant falls during the *Black Death* (1348–9) pandemic and the *Industrial Revolution*. But the same cannot be concluded about weight! Perhaps the best known of relatively recent examples is the following. In January 2014, London's *The Daily Telegraph* newspaper published an article: '*Why are we fatter than ever?*' It began with reference to an advertisement in the London *Times* over two centuries previously – on 2 April 1806 – indicating that for an admission fee of one shilling, an observer could at first hand see 'the greatest curiosity in the world'. The writer was referring to a man, Daniel Lambert (1770–1809), who at 36 years weighed more than 50 stone (>317 kg) and was one of Leicester's 'most cherished icons' (*see* fig 0.1); some three years later he was dead! In his youth he had been 'fit and strong', and on one occasion was reputed to have fought a bear in a street (presumably in Leicester)! It was only after he transferred to a *sedentary* occupation, as a Leicester gaolkeeper, that he 'dramatically gained weight'. Today, the article continued, he would have been 'in need of [i] a triple-width aircraft seat and [ii] a wardrobe-sized coffin'; 'We Brits are fatter and heavier than ever before in history ...'.

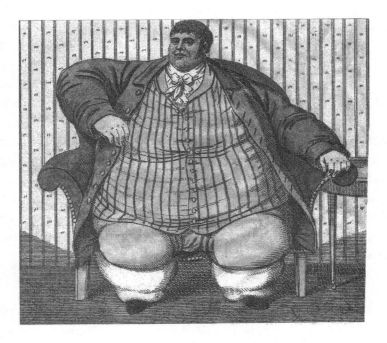

Fig 0.1: Daniel Lambert of Leicester –in 1809. (*Daily Telegraph, Lond* 2014; 6 January: 25.)

While in former times it was [primarily] the rich who were at risk, now ... obesity is unequivocally linked to poverty ...'. 'In the past [we are told] the person with [a] feeble appetite would be the one who died in winter [whereas today] food is not only constantly available [but both] plentiful and ... cheap'. Whereas one hundred years ago, 'up to 70 per cent of [an] average income went on food, today that figure is only about 10 per cent of [an] average earnings, excluding alcohol'. Furthermore, meals are now 'easy, convenient and [possess] a long shelf life', this change has come about largely because wives and other women spend most of their day in the workplace. As a consequence, 'manufacturers [have] added sugar and fat to … highly processed food [in order] to make it [more] palatable.' In former days, 'If you were hungry … between meals, you ate an apple or a slice of bread; chocolate being reserved for special occasions. Today, with food available all day [and] every day, we snack at will on calorie-dense soft drinks, savouries, pasties and choc-chip biscuits'. The author of this article quoted an Oxford Professor of *Diet and Population Health* as indicating that 'Now you can get a three-course meal at a petrol station' in contrast to 'a sandwich in a Tupperware box' on a day trip. Whereas some fifty years ago, a typical dinner perhaps consisted of lamb chops and boiled potatoes, but *now* we have 'Indian, Chinese, Mexican and Thai [food] to constantly whet our appetites'. 'Larger plates, cups and portions, especially of ready meals are another factor' in over-consumption of food. Alcohol (as an appetite stimulant) 'may be another factor', as well as present-day 'marketing strategies'. Why can't we exert some willpower and eat less? (she asked); the answer might lie in the '[relatively short length] of time that food has been plentiful [and the fact that] we haven't had a chance to evolve and catch up', coupled with the fact that '… signals of *fullness* are weak'!

Fig 0.2 shows a *Punch* cartoon – dated 1844 – satirising likely consequences of obesity.[8]

A further historical example – this time fictional – was Charles Dickens (1812–70)'s fat boy (Joe) in *Pickwick Papers* (1837) whose '… waking hours [were] devoted to eating and drinking or to mere contemplation of these activities'. Perhaps not everything about being overweight is negative however; a paper in *Psychological Medicine* has, for example, alluded to the fact that, like Dickens, realisation that obese men 'in their prime' are, unlike many underweight young women, happier and 'generally more relaxed about life'.[9]

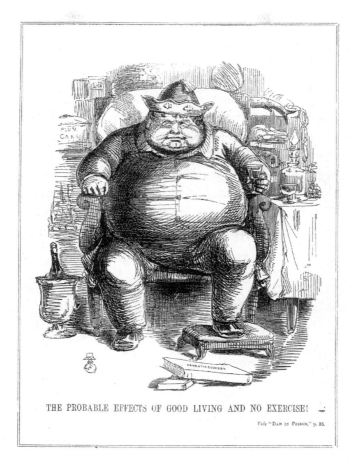

THE PROBABLE EFFECTS OF GOOD LIVING AND NO EXERCISE!

Vide "DAN IN PRISON," p. 38.

Fig 0.2: Mid-nineteenth century cartoon indicating some adverse effects of obesity. (*Punch or the London Charivari* 1844; 21: 38.)

Pathophysiology of obesity

Much of this book emphasises the rôle of *fructose,* and also an imbalance between intake and output of *calories*, but it should be borne in mind that we now know that the mammalian body possesses *hormonal* factors designed to regulate appetite. *Leptin*, discovered in 1994, and other hormones – acting on the hypothalamus – have been implicated in regulation of both appetite and dietary intake (*see* Chapter 9). While *ghrelin* (produced by the stomach) probably controls *short-term* appetite, *leptin* (essentially under control of adipose tissue) is responsible for *long-term* regulation. Most obese individuals have a high *leptin* concentration but have regrettably become resistant to its influence; therefore, administration of *leptin*, with the aim of appetite suppression, is ineffective in the majority of individuals. *Leptin* deficiency results in excessive food consumption, and could possibly account for some genetic and acquired forms of obesity. An hypothesis based on qualitative differences in colonic flora between lean and obese individuals has also evolved; while this might be relevant to metabolic potential in some, it remains unclear as to whether this is causative or possesses a resultant rôle in obesity.[10]

On a negative tack, evidence of smuggling of '*refined-sugar*' by Kenyan troops in Somalia has recently emerged. Taxes raised from this particular scam are estimated to amount to $400 million annually.[11]

What to do?
It is therefore clear that significant changes in lifestyle (including regulation of both dietary components as well as increased exercise (*see* Chapter 12) are required as a matter of urgency in order to counteract this major *twenty-first* century human crisis.

An injection to *cure* obesity has stimulated interest, but unfortunately this is some way off and would be of value only in a small proportion of those with a BMI >30. The focus would be on gene(s) implementing fat deposition rather than energy production.[12] Simple reduction in food intake is unfortunately *not* the answer – which was suggested 100 years ago in another context – to this complex matter.[13]

According to one columnist, writing in London's *Sunday Times* newspaper, obesity has cost the *National Health Service* between an estimated £27bn and £46bn, or £5.1bn annually. Also, *type-2-diabetes*, often a complication of obesity costs the NHS £8.8bn annually. When David Cameron (1966–present) resigned as Prime Minister following the European referendum in June 2016, he left plans to combat childhood obesity – especially *advertising* and *promotion* of sugary foods; this was designed to be part of his legacy. When Theresa May (1956–present) took over, a first priority was to erase 24 of 37 pages of this 'national mission (*see* fig 0.3)'.[14] Apart from sheer spite, it is difficult to comprehend the reasoning behind May's actions. This article was supported by one from Jamie Oliver – a high-profile chef – in the same issue of that newspaper which also found May's strategy 'indefensible.'[15] It is to be hoped that the impact on voting at the next parliamentary election will consequently be devastating to the Conservative party! This simply demonstrates once again that present-day politicians (May in particular) have *no* interest in the health of their country's citizens!

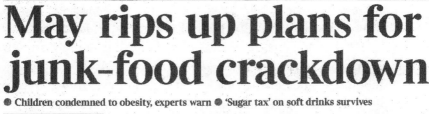

May rips up plans for junk-food crackdown

● Children condemned to obesity, experts warn ● 'Sugar tax' on soft drinks survives

Chris Smyth Health Editor

Tough measures to tackle obesity have been axed after Theresa May overruled

also reacted with outrage at the move. A push by Jeremy Hunt, the health secretary, for "draconian" action was rejected by No 10. It is understood that

ill health. A third of children are too fat, with obesity doubling the risk of early death through conditions ranging from heart disease to cancer.

year of delays, with measures to force companies to take action removed and the industry merely "challenged" not to push junk food to children. Under Mrs

Fig 0.3: Newspaper headline of an article indicating that the incoming British Prime Minister had discarded the initiatives of her predecessor in dealing with the country's *obesity crisis*. (*Times, Lond* 2016; August 18: 1, 2.)

References and notes

1 D Aune, A Sen, M Prasad, T Norat, I Janszky, *et al.* Body mass index and mortality: patterns and paradoxes. *Br med J* 2016; 353 (May 7): 228.

2 *Ibid.*

3 M McCarthy. The jousting accident that turned Henry VIII into a tyrant. *Independent, Lond* 2009: April 17; D Sanderson. Knights want the chance to joust for gold at Olympics. *Times, Lond* 2016; July 21: 9; Anonymous. Joust the ticket; knights in shining armour at the Olympics? Never say never. *Ibid* 2016; July 21: 27.

4 T Whipple. For men, history had its highs and lows. *Ibid* 2017; April 15: 3; Anonymous. Skeletal Prowess: we rise and fall according to the temper of the times, walking tall 700 years ago. *Ibid* 2017; April 15: 29.

5 O Moody. Weighty papers spotted obesity problem first. *Ibid* 2015; July 22: 22.

6 Is fat the new normal? *Sunday Times, Lond* 2015; May 24: 18; H Devlin. Fewer calories for longer life. *Times Lond* 2014; April 2: 13; K Lay. Almost all obese people 'are in denial'. *Ibid* 2014; November 14: 33; C Smyth. GPs are reluctant to talk about obesity. *Ibid* 2015; January 13: 10; E Mills. A Behrmann. Doctors avoid telling patients to lose weight. *Ibid* 2017; February 25: 20; M Porter. No offence intended: doctors need to treat weight gain more seriously. *Times 2, Lond* 2017; February 28: 7.

7 B Lagan. Apple a day does keep doctors away. *Ibid* 2016; April 11: 35; R Blakely. An apple a day: healthcare app will alert doctors to users' weight issues. *Times, Lond* 2014; June 3: 45; T Whipple. Fitness apps are step in wrong direction for health. *Ibid* 2017; February 21: 19; Anonymous. Fit for Purpose: staying healthy is always about taking the first step. *Ibid* 2017; February 21: 29.

8 E Knowles (ed). *The Oxford Dictionary of Quotations* 5th ed. Oxford: Oxford University Press 1999: 905.

9 C Hicks. Why are we fatter than ever? *Daily Telegraph*, London 2014: 6 January: 25–6.

10 C Dickens. *The Posthumous Papers of the Pickwick Club*. London: Chapman and Hall 1837: 607; N Bentley, M Slater, N Burgis. *The*

Dickens Index. Oxford: Oxford University Press 1988: 135; M Wade. Dickens was right: fat men are the happiest. *Times, Lond* 2014; September 6: 34; H Devlin. Dieting may make you healthier, but not happier. *Ibid* 2014; August 7: 15; O Moody. Fatter folk are happier in themselves (so go on, have another mince pie) *Ibid* 2017; December 23: 3.

11 J Leake. Fast food kills bugs that keep you thin. *Sunday Times, Lond* 2015; May 10: 10; T Whipple. Junk food kills bugs that fight illness. *Times, Lond* 2015; May 11; 4; O Moody. Western diet destroys healthy bacteria. *Ibid* June 4: 14; O Moody. Bacteria found in thin people could help to fight obesity. *Ibid* June 15: 20; P Bee. Gut instinct: do you have the right bacteria? It's the new A-list craze that claims the secret to weight-loss lies in your stomach. *Times 2, Lond* 2015; July 28: 6–7.

12 J Starkey. Kenyan troops run $400m sugar scam. *Times, Lond* 2015; November 13: 43.

13 N Badshah. Jab brings hope of cure for obesity. *Ibid* 2015; August 20: 19. (*See also*: O Moody. Injection could help to burn away the fat. *Ibid* 2016; July 1: 24.)

14 Anonymous. On this day: we must eat less. *Ibid* 2017; February 17: 28.

15 T Rayment. May takes bite out of child obesity fight. *Sunday Times, Lond* 2016; October 30: 12.

16 J Oliver. May's child obesity plan is all flab and no meat. *Times, Lond* 2016; October 30: 28.

Part I:

The quest for sweetness and frequency of obesity

CHAPTER 1:

The obesity pandemic: extent of the problem in Britain and its consequences

Only a small percentage of the British population regards obesity as being a *healthy* state.[1] To the vast majority this, together with its numerous complications, denotes a serious *disease*. Striking headlines in contemporary British newspapers include the following: '**75% of British men will be obese by 2030**'. '**Hospitals admit 300,000 obese women in in one year**', '**Britain, the fat man of Europe**', and '**Sweet-toothed Britain is named and shamed**'.[2]

Is obesity a new disease?

It is impossible to accurately document the frequency of being overweight or obese in former ages, but it seems likely that only rich and aristocratic individuals were involved, and this probably only applied in the 'western world'. In an attempt to answer this question, a group of American academics analysed 52 famous paintings of Jesus Christ's Last Supper in western European art galleries and reported their findings in the *International Journal of Obesity:* images indicate that appetite and calorie intake of the Apostles have become 'increasingly prodigious' throughout the ages, suggesting that the present 'obesity epidemic' might have 'deep historical roots'. Overeating has thus undergone a 'general trend [upwards during at least] the last millennium' – which has evolved in the minds of the *artists* rather than their original subjects![3] The last 1,000 years have seen dramatic developments in availability, safety, and abundance of food, despite the fact that according to some 'experts', the present obesity *epidemic* only began 40–50 years ago. It is however, difficult to accept at face value the accuracy of an artist's depiction of the human body. As an example, in a debate – *Body Image* – which focused on the artist's work as an example of power, lust, compassion, elegance, poetry and violence, Germaine Greer (1939–present) a feminist and emeritus Professor of English at Warwick University, has highlighted the fact that

Peter Paul Rubens (1577–1640) painted 'fat' women exclusively.[4] Later, during the Great War (1914–18), a British prisoner-of-war, who clearly possessed well developed artistic talents, depicted in a painting which was exhibited by the *National Army Museum,* one of his (German) guards as a man with a huge 'beer belly' (*see* fig 1.1).[5]

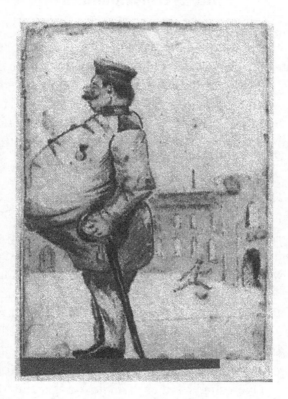

Fig 1.1: Cartoon drawn in 1914–18 depicting a German guard at a POW camp – showing a huge 'beer-belly'. *Times, Lond* 2015; March 7: 16.

Is income a major factor?

Being overweight is obviously *not* at present a class-associated disease; that obesity is not confined to poorer classes is borne out by a contemporary Belgian general medical practitioner, who later became the country's health minister, and who is grossly overweight (*see* fig 1.2); however, appointing a 20-stone woman to this prestigious position has apparently divided the national government! Another recent example is a grossly obese couple who married at the taxpayer's expense (*see* Chapter 2).[6] Now that individuals in the 'Third World' frequently eat in both quality and quantity in a way similar to people in the 'west', obesity there is also becoming commonplace; for example, both South Africa and Mexico now have obesity-rates which are even higher than those in Britain – 66 and 68% respectively, and it is estimated that almost one billion people in *developing* countries are now either overweight or obese.[7]

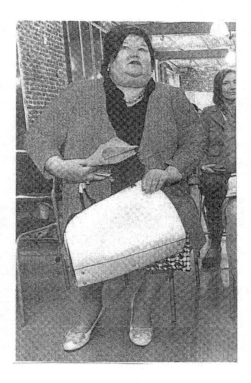

Fig 1.2: Photograph of the Belgian health minister; an example of obesity in an affluent class. *Times, Lond* 2014; October 16: 44.

Obesity – a major problem in present-day Britain!
No less a body than the *World Health Organisation* (WHO) has concluded that *Homo sapiens* is currently ingesting far too much '*refined-sugar*'. In January 2014, the *Times* newspaper published on its front page in bold capitals, a banner headline: Britain's obesity crisis: time for shock

tactics (*see* fig 1.3). Beneath this was the sub-title, 'Treat weight gain like [cigarette] smoking, doctors urged'. This article, by the newspaper's Health Correspondent, referred to a 'domesday scenario' when at least half the inhabitants of Britain will be obese. He quoted the *National Obesity Forum* (NOF), which had recently recommended that 'weight must be confronted like smoking, with children converted to healthy living at a young age'. The *National Health Service* (NHS), he wrote, 'needs to offer better weight-loss programmes if the country is not in future to be crippled by cancer, heart disease, diabetes [all complications of obesity – *see* Chapter 11] and other weight-related [problems] ...'.[8] By the time of that publication, in early 2014, the Chairman of NOF had already indicated that 'A *quarter* of adults [were] already obese [while] two-thirds [weighed] too much', and further that Britain was 'falling behind the [USA] in improving diets'. The forum placed a great deal of responsibility on 'health professionals, a number of whom apparently already have 'weight problems themselves'.[9]

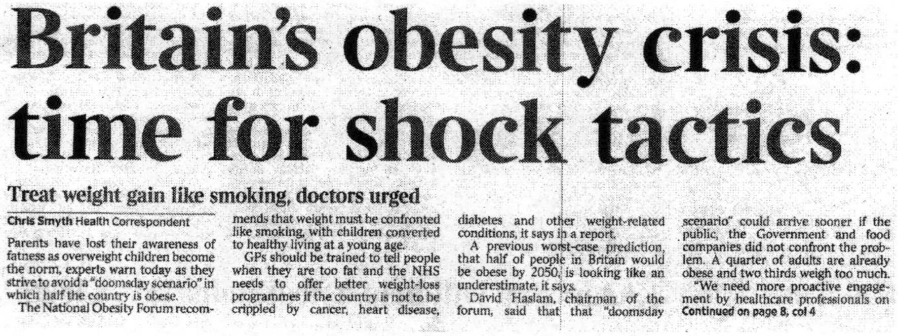

Britain's obesity crisis: time for shock tactics

Treat weight gain like smoking, doctors urged

Chris Smyth Health Correspondent

Parents have lost their awareness of fatness as overweight children become the norm, experts warn today as they strive to avoid a "doomsday scenario" in which half the country is obese.

The National Obesity Forum recommends that weight must be confronted like smoking, with children converted to healthy living at a young age.

GPs should be trained to tell people when they are too fat and the NHS needs to offer better weight-loss programmes if the country is not to be crippled by cancer, heart disease, diabetes and other weight-related conditions, it says in a report.

A previous worst-case prediction, that half of people in Britain would be obese by 2050, is looking like an underestimate, it says.

David Haslam, chairman of the forum, said that that "doomsday scenario" could arrive sooner if the public, the Government and food companies did not confront the problem. A quarter of adults are already obese and two thirds weigh too much.

"We need more proactive engagement by healthcare professionals on Continued on page 8, col 4

Fig 1.3: Headline referring to an article in the London *Times* newspaper (2014 January 13; 1, 8).

Another article indicated that 'Britain is in the bottom 40 [world] countries ... as far as obesity rate is concerned, and ... far below France, Switzerland and Italy', the situation being even worse in England, Scotland, Wales and also Northern Ireland. Also, 'Nearly two thirds of British adults are overweight. When complications of obesity are taken into account, the cost to the NHS in a conservative estimate is £5 billion per year. Legislation (in 2014), public education [and] self-regulation by the food industry' have all failed to improve the situation (*ie,* a balance between calories consumed and those expended), is yet to be achieved, but 'what we choose to buy and eat' must remain a personal matter. The article concluded that time for 'a [much] tougher rôle [of] government has been reached'. However, 'local responses are often more effective than national ones'; in Coventry (England) and Oklahoma City (USA), where weight-loss crusades have been launched, results have been encouraging. Also addressed in the piece was the world scenario; since 1980, in which 'the proportion of overweight or obese children (*see* Chapter 3) rose by 47 per cent ...'. The article concluded that '... Britain is more than ever a nation of couch potatoes'.[10]

ARMED SERVICES

Two other newspaper articles targeted alarming rates of obesity in the army – *'British troops too fat to fight'* (*see* fig 1.4) and *'Army battle of bulge sparks dessert storm'* (*see* fig 1.5). The former was accompanied by another *'Ready, aim, bin the chips, Private Fattie'* (*see* fig 1.6). Thousands of troops were considered 'not fit enough to perform the mandatory number of press-ups and sit-ups' while over 32,000 soldiers had failed a basic fitness test. Affected soldiers were also judged to be 'at increased risk of type-2-diabetes, high blood pressure, and heart disease ...' (*see* Chapter 11). A particular problem apparently existed in Scottish infantry regiments, *eg,* the *Royal Regiment of Scotland,* members of which had 'failed fitness tests 630 times in the past three years', putting blame on the fact that 'military canteen food' was responsible; this problem applied to both male and female military personnel.[11] A later article by the same authors indicated that 'Dozens of [British] servicemen [had already been] discharged for obesity'; again, a poor diet was blamed as the overwhelming culprit.[12]

British troops too fat to fight

Sean Rayment and Mark Hookham

THE British Army appears to be losing the Battle of the Bulge after figures revealed thousands of troops were not fit enough to perform the mandatory number of press-ups and sit-ups.

More than 32,000 soldiers have failed a basic fitness test, which also includes a timed run, at some point during the past three years.

One officer blamed an "appalling diet", which for troops at Camp Bastion in Afghanistan has included a daily cooked breakfast, a cheeseboard, pizza and choice from an extensive dessert buffet boasting profiteroles, ice-cream and cheesecake.

Professor David Haslam, chairman of the National Obesity Forum, said the figures, revealed by a freedom of information request, were "shocking". "I would have

thought it was the job of the army to keep them fit under all circumstances, and if they are not fit, to get them fit," he said.

All soldiers in the army, including senior officers, are expected to undergo a basic fitness test twice a year.

Figures showed 29,600 servicemen and 2,819 female troops failed the test at some point between April 2011 and March 2014.

Ready, aim, bin the chips, page 9

Fig 1.4: Title to an article in the London *Sunday Times* in 2014 (June 22: 1).

Army battle of bulge sparks dessert storm

Billy Kenber

More than 32,000 British Army soldiers have failed a basic fitness test in the past three years amid concerns that military canteen food is taking its toll.

ness assessment involves completing a 1½-mile run in 10½ minutes for men and 13 minutes for women. Soldiers are also expected to manage 50 sit-ups in two minutes, with men also doing 44 press-ups in the same time period and

Fig 1.5: Headline referring to an article in the London *Times* in 2014 (June 23: 15)

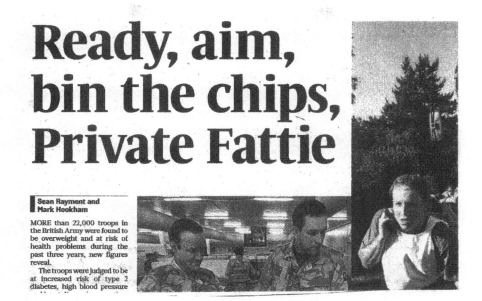

Ready, aim, bin the chips, Private Fattie

Sean Rayment and
Mark Hookham

MORE than 22,000 troops in
the British Army were found to
be overweight and at risk of
health problems during the
past three years, new figures
reveal.
The troops were judged to be
at increased risk of type 2
diabetes, high blood pressure

Fig 1.6: Title to an article in the London *Sunday Times* (2014; June 22: 9).

In reality, obesity has become so common in Britain, that a recent article claimed that it is a greater burden than terrorism, and meanwhile creates an annual loss amounting to 3% of our GDP. Obesity in fact costs the economy a total of £47 billion annually. In 2012, 'impact of smoking on the economy' (the greatest challenger to obesity) was estimated at £57 billion. The answer, in the opinion of this writer, is to:

- Improve and standardise school meals,
- Remove snacks from supermarket checkouts,
- Make bariatric surgery (*see* Chapter 15) more readily available,
- Ban vending machines from schools, and
- Improve nutritional information on food packaging.

In addition, more bicycling should be strongly encouraged.[13]

In another assessment, Britain was placed 111 out of 133 countries compared by their obesity levels; 25% of the British population was declared overweight, compared with 15.6% in France, 17.2% in Italy and 21.3% in Germany.[14] In an accompanying leading article, entitled '*Eat*

Less' the main focus was on complications, headed by diabetes mellitus. Over the last century, the article continued, the trend in health-care has been on increased longevity (which in South Korea has already reached an average of 90 years), but owing to a poor diet, this outcome is now in danger of being *reversed*. In the *nineteenth* century, an emphasis on *public health* was on control of infectious disease; now, the major strategy is to reduce obesity – which, with a more affluent and sedentary population is far more difficult.[15]

An article based on a WHO projection, published a 'league table' of rates of males overweight or obese throughout Europe: in 2010 the UK was ranked fourth (with a rate of 70%) – Ireland, Malta and Iceland were above; UK females (with a rate of 59%) did slightly better, falling fifth – below Belgium, Bulgaria, Russia and Turkey. The prediction from that forecast was that 'by the end of this decade' (*ie*, 2020) the situation across Europe will be far worse, but the UK might fare marginally better! European rates for obesity by 2030 were predicted to undergo a rise to 36% in men, and 33% for women. Despite the fact that increased consumption of salt and fat occurs in Holland compared with the UK, bicycling is more common and as a consequence rates of being either overweight or obese are significantly lower.[16] It is probably also important to delineate precisely *where* fat has accumulated; deposition 'around the waist' (*ie,* 'beer belly') probably predicts an early grave.[17] The waistline of Britain's teenage girls has been the subject of comment in a study conducted at *Leeds Metropolitan University* and published in *Public Health*. By the age of sixteen, 60% of girls were obese, and in two decades (*ie,* 1990–2010), the waistline of the average 15-year-old British schoolgirl expanded by almost 13 cm (five inches). Because increased fat is largely deposited around the waist, this would *not* be reflected in the BMI (*see* Prologue)![18]

Ethnicity

A report from the *Office for National Statistics* indicated that, perhaps surprisingly, unlike health problems previously investigated, which presumably included obesity, it was twice as common in Britain's white, compared with black and Asian communities, this result being attributed to a 'poor diet' together with 'higher levels of [alcohol] consumption'.[19]

Effect of obesity on longevity

Some are, therefore, of the view that overeating is disastrous as far as longevity is concerned, and that everyone is ingesting far too much. In the largest worldwide study devoted to an association between calories and longevity, carried out by researchers at Oxford, Cambridge and Harvard Universities, and reported in the *Lancet*, predictability of premature death in obese individuals was followed (*see* table 1.1). The *conclusion* was that obesity actually reduces life-expectancy (usually from its complications), but much more markedly in men than women. Furthermore, average weight of Britons has steadily risen since 1970, and currently 61% of adults are either overweight or obese, representing an average rise of 1.5 kg each decade.[20]

Table 1.1: Predictability of premature death – in relation to BMI*

BMI (kg m²)	Risk of premature death (%) compared with those of normal weight	
	Men	Women
15–18.5	83	53
18.5–25	0	0
25–30	12	8
30–35	70	37
35–40	268	186
40–60	424	273

Conclusion

So disastrous is the present *obesity epidemic* in Britain (and throughout the whole world) that in the minds of many it should be treated with urgency, and in a way comparable to that of tobacco smoking. It is a problem affecting both sexes, men apparently being as neurotic as women about being overweight.[21] Another article stressed that advertising campaigns could actually backfire by 'driving overweight people to eat more (as a result of) depression',[22] a theme which was pursued in a report commenting on an article in the journal *Obesity*, in which one health correspondent

---

* *see* ref 20 (Knapton); + normal BMI

concluded that prejudice against overweight and obese individuals is, in fact, comparable to sexism and racism'.[23] Isolated obesity might seem harmless, but its complications (*see* Chapter 11) inevitably arise during the subsequent 20 years, as illustrated in an article in the *Journal of the American College of Cardiology*.[24] Lastly, it must be stressed that obesity, especially in men, can reduce longevity significantly (*see* table 1.1).[25]

References and notes

1   M Bateson. Being overweight is 'good for health'. *Times, Lond* 217; March 10: 32; M Kendrick. Playing the weighting game: researchers have determined that being overweight is healthier – and can lead people to live longer. *Independent, Lond* 2015; April 7: 32–3.

2   O Moody. 75% of British men 'will be obese by 2030'. *Times, Lond* 2014; May 10: 4; K Gibbons. Hospitals admit 300,000 obese women in one year. *Ibid* 2016; April 1: 29; K Gibbons. Britain, the fat man of Europe. *Ibid* 2016; April 1: 4; O Moody. Sweet-toothed Britain is named and shamed. *Ibid* 2016; June 4: 4; V Low. A new level of [royal] protection. *Ibid* 2016; December 8: 21; C Smyth. Fat man of Europe: 63 per cent of British adults are overweight. *Ibid* 2017; November 4:4.

3   C Smyth. Artists reflect the course of obesity with expanding portions in the Last Supper. *Ibid* 2010; March 24: 11.

4   J Malvern. Rubens' larger ladies were not about body image, protests Greer. *Ibid* 2015; January 12: 17.

5   S de Bruxelles. How one PoW mocked guards. *Ibid* 2015; March 7: 16.

6   C Bremner. Obese Belgian GP becomes health minister. *Ibid* 2014; October 16: 44; Anonymous. Obese couple wed at taxpayers' expense. *Ibid* 2015; January 6: 3.

7   C Smyth. Obesity spreads to world's poorest. *Ibid* 2014; January 3: 9; Anonymous. Obesity link to poverty. *Ibid* 2017; January 11: 4; Anonymous. Healthier diet 'cheaper than junk food'. *Ibid* 2014; March 2: 2.

8   C Smyth. Britain's obesity crisis: time for shock tactics. Treat weight gain like smoking, doctors urged. *Ibid* 2014; January 13: 1, 8. (*See also*: P Sever. Our obesity epidemic and the food industry. *Ibid* 2014; January 11: 25.)

9   Anonymous. Fast food fatties: celebrity activism and public education have failed to stop the British eating too much. The result is an epidemic of obesity. *Ibid* 2014; May 29: 24.

10 C Smyth. Obesity crisis could ruin us, NHS boss says. *Ibid* 2015; May 19: 17.

11 S Rayment, M Hookham. British troops too fat to fight. *Sunday Times:*

Lond 2014; June 22: 1; B Kenber. Army battle of bulge sparks dessert storm. *Times, Lond* 2014; June 23; Ready, aim, bin the chips, private fatty. *Sunday Times, Lond* 2014; June 22: 9. (*See also*: 15; W Pavia. Supersized army losing obesity battle. *Ibid* 2016; September 14: 30.)

12 M Hookham, S Rayment. Dozens of servicemen discharged for obesity. *Sunday Times, Lond* 2015; October 18: 7; D Rankin. Marching orders for 28st soldier in war on obesity. *Times, Lond* 2016; October 10: 19.

13 K Burgess. Obesity a bigger economic burden than terror. *Ibid* 2014; November 21: 33.

14 N Woolcock. UK is a nation of fatties at risk from infectious disease. *Ibid* 2015; April 9: 4.

15 Anonymous. Eat Less: Britain is a fine place to live but its population needs to stop the growth of obesity. *Ibid* 2015; April 9: 27; K Lay, R Bennett. Living to 90 will be the new norm. *Ibid* 2017; February 22: 9; (*See also*: G C Cook. *Health and sanitation in Victorian Britain: lessons for the 'Third World'*. Ely, Cambridgeshire: Melrose Books 2015: 302.)

16 C Smyth. We may be getting fatter, but not as fast as rest of Europe. *Times, Lond* 2015: May 6: 6.

17 T Whipple. Roll of fat around the waist doubles risk of an early death. *Ibid* 2015; November 10: 1, 6.

18 C Smyth. Sixty per cent of girls obese by 16, says new waistline measure. *Ibid* 2013; November 26: 18.

19 R Bennett. White people suffer most from ill health. *Ibid* 2014; April 2: 5.

20 T Whipple. Secret of long life is 1,500 calories a day. *Ibid* 2017; January 18: 5; S Knapton. Obese people can lose years off their lives – and men are in greater danger: study shows weight of average person has risen 3lbs every decade since 70s. *Daily Telegraph, Lond* 2016; July 14: 15. (*See also*: Anonymous. Obesity risk to man. *Times, Lond* 2016; July 14: 18; O Moody. Obese people who shed pounds will still die early. *Ibid* 2016; January 5: 12; O Moody. Being overweight ages the brain by a decade. *Ibid* 2016; August 5: 16; S Bailey. Obesity and health. *Ibid* 2016 August 20: 26.)

21 C Smyth. Britain's obesity crisis: time for shock tactics: treat weight

gain like smoking, doctors urged. *Ibid* 2014; January 13: 1,8.

22 N Hellen. To live a long life, keep your waistline at half your height. *Sunday Times, Lond* 2014; September 7: 7; Anonymous. Weight and waistline angst: why fat is not just a feminist issue. *Times 2, Lond* 2014: September 20: 6–7; T Whipple. Roll of fat around the waist doubles risk of an early death. *Times, Lond* 2015; November 10: 1, 6; C Smyth. Expanding waist? Blame noisy traffic. *Ibid* 2015; May 26: 2; K Gibbons. Large waists put 92 per cent of women at risk. *Ibid* 2016; December 9: 1, 2.

23 C Smyth. Prejudice against fat people as bad as racism, say scientists. *Ibid* 2014; September 11: 1, 2.

24 Anonymous. Bad news for fat people in good health: it won't last. *Ibid* 2015; January 6: 22.

25 Op cit. *See* note 20 above.

CHAPTER 2:

Social and indirect consequences of being obese

Social consequences both to 'victims' of obesity and those close to them have perhaps in the past been underestimated. In 2014–16, several media articles focused on some of these issues. In fact, it is difficult to avoid the conclusion that the European Court (EC)'s decision (*see* below) possibly swayed opinion which precipitated the momentous verdict for Britain to opt out of that organisation on 23 June 2016!

Is obesity in itself a 'disability'?

A European *Court of Justice* at a Luxembourg meeting in July 2014 (at a time when Britain remained in the *European Union* [EU]), ruled that morbidly obese employees should be provided with larger office seats, lifts and priority parking, as well as special uniforms, etc. This decision, it was said, would apparently affect an estimated one million individuals with a BMI >40 who, under an *Equality* Act of 2010, would in consequence be protected. Although not then law, this ruling was soon due to go before the full European Court (*see* below). It was, however, pointed out that organisations demanding a *fitness* image, such as a health club, etc, would be *seriously* affected.[1] In the same issue of the *Times* newspaper, the writer of the 'Thunderer' column claimed that this decision could lead to obese individuals becoming even fatter, because the former would, by ingesting a 'wrong' diet, strive to become *morbidly* obese with the aim of being categorised as disabled![2] In December 2014, the Court (the highest in the EU) ruled that:

Obesity can be a disability and overweight workers must be protected (by their bosses) from discrimination.

Thus they could *not* be sacked even though the disease was disabling, and could in consequence interfere with employment. This also meant that companies would be *compelled* to provide larger desks and chairs for those 'disabled by … size'. Also, doors might require widening! This ruling could, of course, also lead to employers, when hiring, selecting a slimmer candidate. The article pointed out that in Britain, 6% of adults are already either overweight or obese and therefore should this ruling be accepted, ramifications would be immense. This article was accompanied by another *leading article* which described the ruling as 'a nonsense', the legislation (it claimed) both undermining the 'moral importance of existing anti-discrimination' which would also discourage obese individuals from losing weight. Furthermore, it made claims for 'unfair dismissal' far more likely.[3]

Several days later, this ruling was deemed both 'fatalistic and daft' by the head of the *National Health Service* (NHS).[4] This controversy attracted several letters, also published in the *Times* newspaper; it was pointed out that although '*Morbid Obesity* can certainly debilitate it need not disable *permanently*'. Other correspondence also focused on potential reversibility of obesity, the fact that obesity *per se* does not equate with under-performance, and also the fact that small businesses would be unable, owing to inability to provide extra facilities, to employ anyone who *was* obese.[5]

Consequences of being obese
Obese individuals are frequently 'in denial' or are not aware of the problem(s) (see also: Prologue). Only about one-tenth of clinically obese individuals (11% women and 7% men) in Britain accepted that they possessed a serious weight-problem, according to results of a survey published in *BMJ Open*. Furthermore, only 10% were aware that the BMI obesity threshold is 30, or that they were facing *serious* complications of obesity (*see* Chapter 11).[6] A further problem is that general practitioners (GPs) are frequently reluctant to indicate to their patients that they are either overweight or obese (*see* Prologue). In a study at King's College London, and also reported in *BMJ Open*, only 20% of obese patients had previously received either dietary advice or anti-obesity drugs from their GP. In those who were already *morbidly* obese, no less than 41% were in that category.[7]

Employment and obesity

A report in a *Times 2* supplement indicated that difficulty in finding employment associated with obesity is often caused by the fact that obese people are frequently subjects of abuse. If they are both abused *and* also found to be disabled they are probably legally immune and should get office protection under the *Equality* Act (2010) (*see* above).[8]

Pay and benefits for obese individuals

The 'drain' on Britain's economy (cost of drugs was considered significant) posed by the obesity *epidemic* and its consequences was the subject of a government review in 2015. The cost to the NHS was estimated to be >£5 billion, and individually £27 annually; this included compensation for illness for days lost at work as well as for welfare. If treatment is refused, benefits are at risk! Already, fatter and shorter staff are paid significantly less, but they are generally from a lower social stratum, and have had a poorer education and nutritional background.[9]

Financial penalties for the obese

Loss of benefits for the obese had also been suggested by the previous British Prime Minister – David Cameron. Such a ruling would have put overweight individuals on a level with alcoholics and drug addicts; however, this suggested strategy was therefore forcefully opposed by a significant section of the medical press.[10]

Taxpayers' liability

In January 2015 a couple who claimed to be 'too fat to work' on account of obesity (*see* fig 2.1) because their combined weight was 54 stone (almost 343 kg) were apparently receiving benefits amounting to £2,000 monthly. Furthermore, they had recently married at a taxpayer-funded ceremony which had cost £3,000. The male partner, who of the two was 31 stone (nearly 197kg) and the more obese had previously been married *five* times, and was claimed unsurprisingly to be '*addicted to food*'![11]

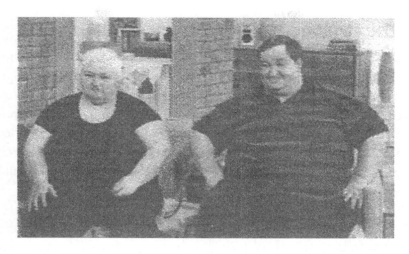

Fig 2.1: An obese married couple (whose respective body weights were 23 and 31 stone) – who claimed tax relief for their weight-related disabilities (*Times, Lond* 2015; January 6: 3.)

Overweight commuters
A female British Member of Parliament – a trained nurse and former health minister – perhaps not surprisingly complained that during a recent rail journey she was seated next to an *overweight* commuter. The outcome of that unfortunate experience was that overweight and obese commuters should be *recommended* to slim![12]

'Fat haters'
Reports also drew attention to 'fat haters' on London's *underground railway*; the latter claiming that they would *not* tolerate such behaviour and that passengers had every right to 'travel with confidence'.[13]

Reusable shopping bags and obesity
Another report in the *Times* newspaper drew attention to a correlation between people who brought their own bags for shopping purposes, and ones more likely to purchase 'junk' foodstuffs![14]

Other obesity-associated matters
Environmental and physiological factors

The fact that impaired cerebral function might occasionally contribute to obesity has recently gained ground. According to an article in *Biological Psychiatry*, women who are 'stressed-out' apparently metabolise fewer calories and hence increase their weight.[15] Also, 'middle-aged spread', a frequent problem – particularly in men – has according to evidence provided in the journal *Endocrinology*, been partly attributed to a decline in cerebral signals (*via* leptin) to decreased appetite and subsequent consequences on metabolism.[16]

NHS implications

An article in London's *Sunday Times* newspaper claimed that an increase in numbers of hospitals was required to deal with the current obesity *epidemic*. Another stressed how 'hundreds of nurses' were being injured during care of overweight and obese patients.

Regarding staffing, one suggestion was that in order to set an example, overweight members of staff should be 'put on a diet'. As far as obese patients are concerned, 'motivational coaching' should be instituted to assist weight-loss and thus avoid diabetes mellitus; however that article continued to indicate that many diets sold to the public are no more than 'money-spinning nutribabble'.[17]

Rescue operations

Implications of obesity on *accessibility* to individuals homes has also been emphasised. For example, firefighters have had to assist removal of fat individuals from their own homes. Windows and even walls have had to be removed![18]

References and notes

1   Anonymous. Substantially Wrong: classifying obesity as a disability is counterintuitive and counterproductive. *Times, Lond* 2014; December 19: 38; F Gibb. Bosses facing a heavy burden as obese are ruled to be disabled. *Sunday Times, Lond* 2014; July 18: 13.

2   R Clark. Europe has given the fat a reason to get even fatter. *Times, Lond* 2014; July 18: 28.

3   F Gibb. Obesity can be disability, European Court decides. *Ibid* 2014; December 19: 13; Op cit *see* note 1 (Anonymous) above.

4   H Line. EU [European Union] obesity ruling is daft, says health chief. *Ibid* 2014; December 27: 31.

5   Correspondence. Is it really right to call obesity a disability? *Ibid* 2014: December 23: 31.

6   K Lay. Almost all obese people 'are in denial'. *Ibid* 2014; November 14: 33.

7   C Smyth. GPs are reluctant to talk about obesity. *Ibid* 2015; January 13: 10.

8   R Crampton. If being fat stops you getting a job it's your own fault. *Times 2, Lond* 2016; April 26: 2; J Leake. Overweight get office protection. *Sunday Times, Lond* 2016; April 24: 8.

9   M Savage. Obese claimants who refuse treatment may be denied benefits. *Times, Lond* 2015; July 29: 15; K Gibbons. Bosses pay shorter and fatter staff less. *Ibid* 2016; March 9: 11.

10   S Coates. Go on a diet or lose your benefits, obese told: drinkers and drug addicts also face clampdown. *Ibid* 2015; February 14: 1, 4; K Lay. Lancet attacks plan to punish obese people. *Ibid* 2015; March 19: 27.

11   Anonymous. Obese couple wed at taxpayers' expense. *Ibid* 2015: January 6: 3. (*See also*: E Fennell. Obesity: one size no longer fits all after European case. *Ibid* 2014; July 24: 50.)

12   G Keate. Fat commuters must slim, says MP. *Ibid* 2014; December 5: 26; J Thalassites. Airline can seat passengers by their weight. *Ibid* 2016; October 25: 23; P Butler. Weighty problem. *Ibid* 2016 October 26: 30. (*See also*: Anonymous. Don't sit down on busy trains if you are fat, commuters told. *Ibid* 2015; March 14: 31; D Habershon. No respite insight for 'fat' commuters. *Ibid* 2014: December 8: 29; M

Hookham. HS2 trains bulk up for the bulky. *Sunday Times, Lond* 2017; April 30: 1.)

13 D Sanderson. Trolls target woman given 'fat-shaming' card on the tube. *Times, Lond* 2015; December 2: 27; S Elks. Woman given 'fat shaming' card on tube. *Ibid* 2015; December 1: 27; D Ross. My card for the fat-haters. *Times 2, Lond* 2015; December 3: 2.

14 K Lay. Why reusable shopping bags make you fat. *Times, Lond* 2015; July 9: 11.

15 C Smyth. Stressed-out women burn fewer calories. *Ibid* 2014; July 14: 17.

16 H Devlin. Blame declining brain power for that middle-aged spread. *Ibid* 2014; August 13: 4.

17 J Ungoed-Thomas. More hospitals needed to cope with obesity. *Sunday Times, Lond* 2015; January 4: 17; Anonymous. Fat suits for medical staff learning to treat obesity. *Times, Lond* 2013; December 31: 15; K Lay. Health chiefs dismiss fad diets as money-spinning 'nutribabble'. *Ibid* 2015; February 16: 23; C Smyth. Overweight NHS staff put on diet to set an example. *Ibid* 2015; March 12: 10; K Lay. NHS motivators will coach fat people on losing weight. *Ibid* 2015: August 27: 26; K Gibbons. Hundreds of nurses injured caring for overweight patients. *Ibid* 2016; June 1: 20; C Smyth. Dance and fitness classes to keep NHS staff healthy. *Ibid* 2016; March 5: 4; C Smyth. Fat nurses make healthy eating tips hard to swallow. *Ibid* 2017; December 5: 11; C Smyth. Hospital bans staff's sugar snacks to inspire patients. *Ibid* 2018, January 9: 6.

18 G Swerling. Thousands of obese people rescued from own houses. *Ibid* 2015; December 29: 5; K Gibbons. Fire crews move obese three times a day. *Ibid* 2016; September 20: 8.

CHAPTER 3:

Special problems in infants and children: the next generation and most vulnerable group

Obviously today's children will become British adults of the next generation, and it is of paramount importance to strive to make them as healthy as possible. A *Times* leading article in 2015 succinctly summarised the present childhood *obesity epidemic* and its potential solution. By age 11 years, one third of children are now overweight or obese, and the solution will lie in a combination of: public education, tax policy, and legislation (*see* Chapter 7). The present situation has in fact already become 'a public health disaster'; overall, 'twice as many Britons [children included] are classified as being obese [which was not the case] twenty-five years ago' (*see* Chapter 1). This article, quite rightly, threw a great deal of blame on parents.[1]

Many cases of obesity thus begin in childhood, and recognition of this fact by both *public health* authorities and government, as well as the likely cause(s), is the main focus of this chapter. Clearly, pre-disposing factors which also apply to adults – highlighted in Chapter 1 – are also important.

Obesity will send today's children to early grave

Campaigners attack 'couch potato' culture

Fig 3.1: Principal banner headline on the front page of the London *Times* newspaper in 2013 – August 13: 1.

In late 2013 a *Times* main banner headline declared: **Obesity will send today's children to early grave** (*see* fig 3.1); 'millions of children [the article clearly considered] were shunning vegetables and also exercise in favour of "fizzy drinks" in front of the television'. Distressing figures were also provided by a joint *British Heart Foundation* and *Oxford University* study. Both schools as well as parents were incriminated in that report, and the situation, according to the paper's correspondent, demanded 'wider cultural shifts'. The problem, although worst among *poorer* children, was also common with middle-class parents, who were in fact doing very little about it![2]

Since the 1950s, most British infants and children have been given breakfast cereals; probably a higher percentage than in any other part of Europe. These cereals possess two undesirable additions – '*refined-sugar*' in the majority of cereals – and *salt* in porridge. As time has progressed, the weight of sucrose has escalated, and since the principal target in the minds of the sugar-industry is the *sweet-toothed* child, this has unquestionably boosted sales! That is undoubtedly a major cause of obesity in children.

IN UTERO RISK

A later article in the same newspaper referred to the fact that 'obesity in childhood' can commence *in utero*; therefore, obese women should reduce their weight *before* becoming pregnant (*see also* Chapter 4).[3] The *British Medical Journal* – focusing on an article in *Diabetologia* which was based on a Swedish study involving 1.2 million children – also reported that maternal obesity in the third trimester of pregnancy is a significant factor in pathogenicity of childhood obesity, whereas *type-2-diabetes mellitus* is a frequent corollary.[4] A warning to obese women of childbearing age has also come from Finland; a project funded by the *European Commission,* has clearly demonstrated that children born to obese mothers are themselves more likely to be overweight. This study was based on 13,000 births in Helsinki in the 1930s and 40s, and has also indicated that mothers who were overweight in late pregnancy gave birth to infants more likely to develop: malignancies, ischaemic cardiac disease and strokes as well as diabetes mellitus. This result might, claimed the researchers, be because obese women ate an excess of saturated fat during pregnancy.[5]

WEIGHT FOLLOWING BIRTH

That newborn children are often overweight is thus undeniable; 'weigh-ins' are not necessary to spot the fat child. Regarding childhood obesity, a representative of *Public Health England* (PHE) claimed that 'What is [viewed] as *normal* has changed over time', and the *Association for the Study of Obesity* has pronounced 'that advertisements for *junk* food should be banned ...', because 'Current regulation [has proved] insufficient to alter an environment that challenges child health'.[6]

Accompanying a piece (based on a *University of Washington* survey which was published in the *Lancet – see* below) entitled: '**British girls become the fattest in Europe**' is a table of overweight girls and boys in European countries (*see* fig 3.2 and table 3.1).[7] Apparently one-quarter of 'poor' 10 and 11-year-old children are now obese, and the position is rapidly worsening. These figures are based on *Health and Social Information* statistics – which emanated from state school reception classes in socially 'deprived parts of the country', including Hackney and Southwark.[8]

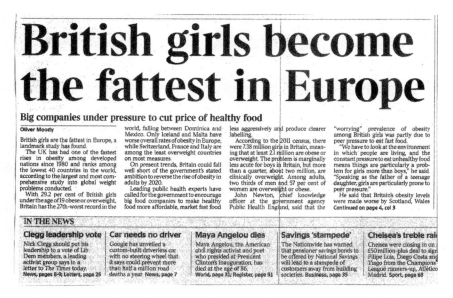

British girls become the fattest in Europe

Big companies under pressure to cut price of healthy food

Oliver Moody

British girls are the fattest in Europe, a landmark study has found.

The UK has had one of the fastest rises in obesity among developed nations since 1980 and ranks among the lowest 40 countries in the world, according to the largest and most comprehensive study into global weight problems conducted.

With 29.2 per cent of British girls under the age of 19 obese or overweight, Britain has the 27th-worst record in the world, falling between Dominica and Mexico. Only Iceland and Malta have worse overall rates of obesity in Europe, while Switzerland, France and Italy are among the least overweight countries on most measures.

On present trends, Britain could fall well short of the government's stated ambition to reverse the rise of obesity in adults by 2020.

Leading public health experts have called for the government to encourage big food companies to make healthy food more affordable, market fast food less aggressively and produce clearer labelling.

According to the 2011 census, there were 7.38 million girls in Britain, meaning that at least 2.1 million are obese or overweight. The problem is marginally less acute for boys in Britain, but more than a quarter, about two million, are clinically overweight. Among adults, two thirds of men and 57 per cent of women are overweight or obese.

John Newton, chief knowledge officer at the government agency Public Health England, said that the "worrying" prevalence of obesity among British girls was partly due to peer pressure to eat fast food.

"We have to look at the environment in which people are living, and the constant pressure to eat unhealthy food means things are particularly a problem for girls more than boys," he said.

"Speaking as the father of a teenage daughter, girls are particularly prone to peer pressure."

He said that Britain's obesity levels were made worse by Scotland, Wales Continued on page 4, col 3

IN THE NEWS

Clegg leadership vote	Car needs no driver	Maya Angelou dies	Savings 'stampede'	Chelsea's treble rai
Nick Clegg should put his leadership to a vote of Lib Dem members, a leading activist group says in a letter to The Times today. News, pages 8-9; Letters, page 25	Google has unveiled a custom-built driverless car with no steering wheel that it says could prevent more than half a million road deaths a year. News, page 7	Maya Angelou, the American civil rights activist and poet who presided at President Clinton's inauguration, has died at the age of 86. World, page 31; Register, page 51	The Nationwide has warned that pensioner savings bonds to be offered by National Savings will lead to a stampede of customers away from building societies. Business, page 35	Chelsea were closing in on £50 million-plus deal to sign Filipe Luis, Diego Costa and Tiago from the Champions League runners-up, Atlético Madrid. Sport, page 68

Fig 3.2: Banner headline in the London *Times* newspaper in 2014 – May 29: 1.

Table 3.1: Percentages of overweight girls and boys (under 20 years) in various European countries[†] (*see also* ref 7)

Country	Girls	Boys
Austria	16.3	18.9
Denmark	19.4	19.7
Finland	21.1	26.0
France	16.0	19.9
Germany	19.4	20.5
Greece	29.1	33.7
Iceland	23.0	26.4
Ireland	26.5	26.6
Italy	24.3	29.9
Malta	25.3	33.6
Netherlands	16.1	18.3
Norway	16.0	20.1
Portugal	27.1	28.7
Spain	23.8	27.6
Sweden	19.3	20.4
Switzerland	16.2	20.7
United Kingdom	29.2	26.1

Another report, in the *Archives of Diseases of Childhood*, also claimed that at least one-third of British children are now either overweight or obese; this was considered to be part of a trend – which bears signs of beginning to plateau – that was in the opinion of 'many parents and children' *not* however of 'serious health concern'.[9] Others claim however that on the contrary, this finding *is* of *major* importance, and it is high time to be judgemental and act accordingly, otherwise these children will become obese adults. The writer of that report referred to George Orwell (1903–50) who, in the 1940s, claimed that 'the poor will always prefer a bit of something "tasty" to [more] healthy options'. However, those who choose to become vegetarians (especially girls) are facing other serious problems.[10]

† *Sunday Times, Lond* 2015 ; May 24 : 17.

PRE-PUBERTAL CHILDREN

A later *Times* first leading-article concentrated on improvements in the diet of Britain's schoolchildren. It blamed the present '... "food environment"' of ubiquitous, cheap fast-food [but probably more importantly] effective *advertising*'. 'While obesity among girls [it continued] is the worst in Europe [*see* above], that among boys is not much better'.[11]

A diagnosis of obesity is usually made very early in life. Babies who are likely to become obese can apparently be recognised when only *six* months old; BMI and readings taken between two and six months being predictive of later obesity.[12] Another report indicated that the number of 12-year-olds weighing >15 stone (95 kg) doubled in 2015, while ⅓ of children leave primary school either overweight or obese.[13] However, another study predicted more encouraging results; although childhood obesity remains a problem, fewer four-year-olds were apparently obese in 2015, and in 11-year-olds that has begun to decline, although obesity remains far more common in the poorer classes.[14] Although biochemical tests for hypothyroidism often gave positive results, it is probable that most are a *consequence* rather than cause of obesity, and most normalise following weight-loss.[15]

While children's '*refined-sugar*' intake has been estimated by some to be *three* times too high, some pupils are apparently still being taught that certain sugary drinks – such as *Coca-Cola* – are *essential* components of a balanced diet.[16] Eating 'unhealthy' food is not, of course, always an individual's choice. Rising costs, together with stagnant wages have meant that many families have had to raise children on cheap but nutritionally 'empty' meals; that is where 'fizzy' drinks and 'sugary' foods enter the scenario, largely because fresh fruit and vegetables are far more expensive. As a result, according to the *Times* health correspondent, the 'spectre of Oliver Twist has returned to Britain', and many children are either permanently hungry or are relatively malnourished.[17] Another columnist has accused both politicians and general practitioners of turning a 'blind eye' to the present childhood *obesity crisis*, which she likened to a Grimm's fairy tale, in which Hansel and Gretel were force-fed by a witch in order to fatten them up prior to their premature demise.[18]

The *Royal College of General Practitioners* has apparently at last recognised that the childhood obesity epidemic is in danger of 'destroying the health of a whole generation of children'. When children commence primary school, nine per cent are obese, and by completion of education that has risen to an average of 19 per cent! The College gave, as an example, an obese seven-year-old child with *type-2-diabetes*. There is also evidence that risk of heart disease is exacerbated by sugary drinks. The author of the article declared, 'We [now] have a generation of patients [children] who may predecease their parents'.[1] The problem of bringing obesity to wider attention and alert parents to risks of the present health crisis has also exerted media thoughts. An extreme measure would involve schools being ranked (graded) by numbers of overweight or obese pupils.[20]

SOLUTION TO THE CHILDHOD OBESITY EPIDEMIC (*SEE ALSO* PART III)
Dietary
An ideal solution to the present obesity epidemic in childhood would be to reduce '*refined-sugar*' consumption, especially that in 'fizzy drinks'. But this is 'easier said than done' as the author of an article in early 2014 indicated; why, she asked, does the *World Health Organisation* (WHO) recommend that only *ten* or possibly *five* per cent of calories (or five teaspoonfuls daily) should consist of '*refined-sugar*?' If it is that bad (she was comparing the situation with tobacco which causes bronchial carcinoma) why not eliminate it from the diet altogether? There is clearly no doubt that '*refined-sugar*' in children's breakfast cereals must be reduced; this targeting of a vulnerable group with this form of 'sweetness' is totally unacceptable. Surely it is time that the British government put an end to destruction of an entire generation, so as to placate sugar industrialists![21] '*refined-sugar*' content of some common breakfast cereals is shown in Chapter 7.

Claims of 'grossly misleading information on packaging', have been made concerning fruit-snacks targeted at children, who are clearly the major recipients. Such products contain more '*refined-sugar*' than a packet of sweets; in fact some consist of 'more than two thirds sugar'. The charity *Action on Sugar* has called on government to reduce this burden on the *National Health Service* (NHS) and *force* the food-industry to 'cut the sugar in its products'. A spokesman for the former British prime minister – David Cameron – was however reported as saying that in 2015 the government was 'inclined to carry on "working with the industry" on a voluntary basis'.[22]

An alternative strategy would be to restrict, or completely ban to children sales of sweet or 'fizzy' drink. While less than one-third of *adults* living in *European Union* (EU) countries consume 'energy drinks', apparently over two-thirds of *adolescents* do![23] Another study has indicated that several energy drinks, including *Lucozade*, contain huge amounts of '*refined-sugar*' – in some as much as twenty teaspoons (78g) are contained in a 500ml can; the authors concluded that such drinks should be banned. Yet another solution would be to remove sweets and chocolates and replace them with 'healthier products' at supermarket 'checkouts'.[24]

Other dietary approaches to the dilemma have also received attention. In a Norwegian study involving 8,000 children aged 11 years in eight European countries, those who ate lunch with their parents were more likely than those who took breakfast and dinner together to be either overweight or obese. The reason for this is unclear![25]

Exercise

Lack of exercise has of course also been incriminated as a major factor in the *obesity epidemic* in childhood. In a survey of 15 countries – including the USA, Scotland, England, Nigeria, Mexico, Australia and New Zealand – published in the *Journal of Physical Activity and Health*, Scottish children were deemed to be the 'laziest in the world', and England was not far behind! Major blame was attributed to new technology – including computer games and television.[26] Do away with 'buggies' and get infants and children walking again – which is precisely what children want, according to a *Times* columnist; 'Bodies that evolved to survive the Stone Age' cannot be treated in this way, she wrote; furthermore, 'obesity and inactivity are the "new smoking"'.[27] Another article called for the 'school run' to be abandoned and for children to be compelled to *walk* to school, while parents 'should be forced to park their cars at least half a mile away.[28] Even when not overtly overweight or obese, many children are at present physically unfit, whereas many '[normal-weight] children [she continued] possess far too much fat and *not* enough muscle [as a result of] inactivity levels....'[29]

Other strategies

School lunches have also come in for a great deal of criticism. One school has banned them altogether, while 'fast-food' firms should perhaps be prevented from making school deliveries. However, another article has indicated that because they eat at home during the summer vacation, it is then that children gain most weight![30] Watching television for as little as one hour daily has been shown to predispose five and six-year-old children to being either overweight or obese; it was concluded from an investigation that childhood television viewing should be strictly limited to as little as two hours which is itself almost certainly too much![31]

Insufficient *sleep* is a lifestyle factor which can contribute to obesity (*see* Chapter 9); toddlers who had too little sleep were frequently overweight at *seven* years old, was concluded from a study at the *Massachusetts General Hospital for Children;* the reason remains unclear, but it is suggested that sleep might influence hunger hormones (*see* Chapter 9) and subsequent metabolism; or that children who stay up late are more likely either to partake of an evening snack, or alternatively indulge in a second dinner with their parents.[32] A follow-up letter indicated that so bad is nutritional advice given at most infant schools – some provided by *Ofsted* – that government should urgently intervene.[33]

Better care in the *playground* has also been recommended. A study at *King's College London* and published in *Psychological Medicine* indicated that bullying of seven–11-year-olds at school was likely to have long-lasting psychological consequences – including obesity – in later life.[34]

Childhood obesity in other countries

Britain is by no means alone in the childhood obesity *epidemic*, which has developed into a *pandemic*. The problem also afflicts Middle Eastern children, who as a result of climatic factors, take only limited exercise; furthermore in the Middle East, vast quantities of '*refined-sugar*' are usually consumed in tea or coffee; hence, childhood obesity is common-place. In an attempt to remedy the situation in Dubai (a *United Arab Emirate* country) a weight-losing campaign has been initiated, and children will henceforth be paid *in gold* for weight-loss![35]

An overall strategy

Owing to this continuing disaster which has stricken the whole world, there have been calls for an *overall strategy*. This was in preparation under Cameron, but apparently destroyed by the present prime minister, May![36]

In **conclusion**, there is no doubt that childhood obesity is a multi-factorial problem. Although '*refined-sugar*' is dominant in this equation, public education, parental control, lax policy, legislation, politics, etc[37] and other factors – especially lack of exercise [38] – are also important. The initiative undertaken by Jamie Oliver – a well-respected chef – to involve schools to a far greater extent in campaigns against childhood obesity should be welcomed. Oliver is totally opposed to 'junk food' together with positive governmental influence on the sugar industry (*see* Chapter 7); he has also advocated annual weighing of children at every junior school.[39]

References and notes

1   Anonymous. Fat chance: childhood obesity is an endemic problem that seems to defy most solutions. *Times, Lond* 2015; January 16: 26; C Smyth. Get tough on child obesity, Jamie Oliver urges PM. *Ibid*; July 16: 2; J Maingay *et al*. Obesity crisis. *Ibid* 2017; February 6: 28. (*See also*: T Whipple. Effect of sugar on children is 'parent myth'. *Ibid* 2015; June 8: 9; K Lay. A fifth of children are obese by 14. *Ibid* 2017; December 7: 21.)

2   C Smyth. Obesity will send today's children to early grave: campaigners attack 'couch potato' culture. *Ibid* 2013; August 12: 1, 7; C Smyth. Children weigh in half a stone heavier. *Ibid* 2017: October 11: 16.

3   C Smyth. Obesity strategy 'is failing': problem begins before birth, warns top child doctor. *Ibid* 2015; May 26: 1, 2.

4   Anonymous. Maternal obesity increases risk in offspring, study shows. *Br med J* 350: 5.

5   K Lay. Your unborn child is at risk of disease, obese women warned. *Times, Lond* 2015; February 17: 15.

6   C Midgley. You don't need school weigh-ins to spot fat children. *Times 2, Lond* 2016; January 13: 2; C Smyth. Britain's obesity crisis: time for shock tactics. *Times, Lond*; January 13: 1 and 8.

7   O Moody. British girls become the fattest in Europe: big companies under pressure to cut price of healthy food. *Ibid*; May 29: 1, 4; C Smyth. Sixty per cent of girls obese by 16, says new waistline measure. *Ibid* 2013; November 26: 18. (*See also*: K Gibbons. Affluent girls are more likely to become obese than boys. *Ibid* 2016; October 11: 2.)

8   K Lay. Quarter of poor 11-year-olds are obese. *Ibid* 2014; December 4: 40.

9   K Lay. One third of children are overweight. *Ibid* 2015; January 30: 17; K Lay. Fat teenagers think their weight is normal. *Ibid* 2015; July 10: 14. (*See also*: M Porter. Can you tell if your child is overweight? It's not that easy. *Times 2, Lond* 2015; March 31: 6.)

10 J Boswell, R Lott-Lavigna. Teen vegan girls put health at risk. *Sunday Times, Lond* 2015; October 4: 14; J Turner. Don't condemn five-year-olds to a life of obesity: one in ten children starting school next week will be overweight. Jamie Oliver is right – it's time to get judgemental.

Times, Lond 2013: August 31: 23.

11 Anonymous. Fast food fatties: celebrity activism and public education have failed to stop the British easting too much. The result is an epidemic of obesity *Ibid* 2104; May 9: 24.

12 Anonymous. Obesity is predicted in babies aged six months. *Ibid* 2016: April 2: 27.

13 F Karim. Number of children who weigh above 15 st doubles. *Ibid* 2016; February 22: 6.

14 K Lay. Fewer four-year-olds are tipping scales into obesity. *Ibid* 2015: November 27: 39.

15 U Niranjan, N P Wright. Should we treat subclinical hypothyroidism in obese children? *Br med J* 2016; 352: 450–1.

16 D Hyde. Children's sugar intake is three times too high, data suggest. *Daily Telegraph, Lond* 2015; July 17: 1; K Lay. Daily fizzy drink can add 30% to body fat. *Times, Lond* 2016; January 12: 22; K Gibbons. Children eat twice the safe level of sugar. *Ibid* 2016; September 10: 11; J Ungoed-Thomas, J Stoneman. Pupils taught cola is part of a healthy diet. *Sunday Times, Lond* 2015; May 24: 13. (*See also*: R Ballam. British Nutrition Foundation explains what goes on the 'eatwell' plate. *Ibid* 2015: May 31: 26; B Kenber. Cuts threaten campaign to curb child obesity *Times, Lond* 2016; July 18: 22; K Gibbons. Children swallow bathtub of sugary drinks each year. *Ibid* 2016; November 22: 28; A Ellson. Junk food adverts aimed at children facing total ban. *Ibid* 2016; December 8: 14; Anonymous. Ad Nauseam: online junk food advertisements aimed at children are to be banned. Good. *Ibid* 2016; December 8: 33.)

17 C Smyth. Children going hungry in 'Oliver Twist Britain'. *Ibid* 2014; May 2: 25. (*See also*: R Richardson. *Dickens & the Workhouse: Oliver Twist and the London poor.* Oxford: Oxford University Press 2012: 370.)

18 A Thomson. This grim tale of children fattened up to die: politicians and GPs are turning a blind eye to the obesity epidemic. If we don't act, we're heading for disaster. *Times, Lond* 2015; March 25: 35. (*See also*: E Lucas (ed). *The Fairy tales of the Brothers Grimm.* London: The Folio Society Ltd 2996: 98–107.)

19 S-K Templeton. GPs declare state of emergency over childhood

obesity threat. *Sunday Times, Lond* 2014; August 31: 7; O Moody. Cutting one fizzy drink lowers child heart risk. *Times, Lond* 2015; September 3: 3. (*See also*: T Whipple. Fat eight-year-olds show signs of heart disease. *Ibid* 2015; November 11: 6; K Gibbons. Ditching sugar cuts heart risk. *Ibid* 2016; July 20: 18; K Lay. Fizzy drinks linked to early puberty and breast cancer. *Ibid* 2015 January 28: 24; C Smyth. Scientists puzzled as heavier twins outlast their siblings. *Ibid* 2016; August 2: 7; K Lay. Fast food next for the bin in childhood obesity fight. *Ibid* 2017; August 18: 16.)

20 K Gibbons. Call to rank schools by pupil obesity. *Ibid* 2016; July 8: 9; N Roskilly. Ranking by obesity. *Ibid* 2016; July 9: 24.

21 H Rumbelow. How can you stop your kids from getting caned on sugar? Scientists are recommending we halve our daily sugar intake to just five teaspoons a day. Do they have children? *Times 2, Lond* 2014; January 9: 4–5; G Narwan. Britons given extra sugar in their cereal. *Times, Lond* 2016; November 29: 9; O Kamm. Breakfast cereals have lost their snap, crackle and pop. *Ibid* 2016; December 29: 22; A Ellson. Cereals suffer in the morning dash. *Ibid* 2016; December 29: 14; G Sandeman. Children are eating three cubes of sugar at breakfast. *Ibid* 2017; January 3: 14; C Smyth. 'Bad diet more dangerous to child health than ebola'. *Ibid* 2017; February 15: 6; J Ungoed-Thomas. 'Healthy wholegrain' biscuits and cereals packed with sugar. *Sunday Times, Lond* 2017; February 19: 3. (*See also*: J Ungoed-Thomas. Kellogg's smothers health crisis in sugar. *Ibid* 2017; April 23: 12; W Humphries. Waitrose bans sales of energy drinks to under-16s. *Ibid* 2018; January 5: 23.)

22 O Moody. Fruit snacks aimed at children contain more sugar than sweets. *Times, Lond* 2015; May 29: 17; T Whipple. Restrict sales of energy drink to children. *Ibid* 2014; October 15: 21.

23 K Lay. Energy drink with 20 teaspoons of sugar 'puts children at risk'. *Ibid* 2015; February 26: 23. (*See also*: G Hurst. Energy drinks are causing classroom chaos, warn teachers. *Ibid* 2015; April 6: 14.)

24 J Simpson. Tesco chooses the healthy option and removes sweets at checkouts. *Ibid* 2014; May 22: 4.

25 O Moody. Family lunch raises a child's risk of obesity. *Ibid* 2014; May 31: 34.

26 N Woolcock. Scottish children are 'least active in world'. *Ibid* 2014; May 21: 21. (*See also*: N Badshah. British children among least active in world. *Ibid* 2016; November 21: 4.)

27 J Russell. Beat obesity. Get your child out of that buggy: Fatness and inactivity are condemning our cosseted, sedentary children to an early grave. *Ibid* 2014; June 12: 30.

28 Anonymous. Call for curb on school run to tackle child obesity. *Ibid* 2014; June 7: 9; G Swerling. Teacher goes the extra mile to beat obesity. *Ibid* 2015; September 29: 17.

29 M Roberts. 'British children's lack of fitness is more worrying than obesity'. *Times 2* 2014; August 2: 4–5; G Swerling, N Woolcock. Pupils lapping up their mile a day. *Times, Lond* 2015; October 3: 19.

30 N Woolcock. School bans packed lunches. *Ibid* 2016; June 18: 35; D Stephenson. Fast-food firms must be banned from delivering to schools. *Ibid* 2016; June 23: 28; K Lay. Summer has diet danger for children. *Ibid* 2015: September 17: 17.

31 Anonymous. Daily hour of TV makes children fat. *Ibid* 2015; April 27: 18.

32 H Devlin. Toddlers who don't sleep enough run obesity risk. *Ibid* 2014; May 19: 5. (*See also*: Chapter 9.)

33 J Hooks. Children's nutrition. *Ibid* 2015; May 28: 28.

34 C Smyth. Bullied children are more likely to be battling obesity in middle age. *Ibid* 2015; May 20: 19.

35 L Callaghan. Obese Dubai children trade pound of flesh for gold. *Sunday Times, Lond* 2014; August 10: 25.

36 J R Ashton *et al.* Obesity strategy 'is long overdue'. *Times, Lond* 2016; March 2: 26; P Kumar *et al.* Obesity action plea. *Ibid* 2016; July 8: 34.

37 Op cit. *See* note 1 above.

38 D Green. Burn off the sugar. *Ibid* 2014; June 30: 29.

39 D Sanderson. Jamie fights war on sugar but keeps his diners in the dark. *Ibid* 2015; September 3: 3; S Griffiths. Jamie calls for pupil weigh-ins. *Sunday Times, Lond* 2015; November 29: 24.

CHAPTER 4:

Cause(s) of the pandemic

Assuming obesity has a predominantly dietary origin, *fructose* is the most likely candidate (*see* Chapter 8). However, there are other possible causes – some of which are outlined in this chapter. Individuals in Britain were significantly slimmer some 50 years ago (1974) compared with today – when 70% of 'middle-aged Britons are either overweight or obese' – a figure attributed to *Public Health England* – an organisation directly answerable to the *British Ministry of Health*. But calorie intake, according to several surveys, is now apparently falling. During those 50 years, there is absolutely no doubt that day-to-day exercise amongst other forms of physical activity, plummeted. In consequence, *less calories* are actually required, and 'small changes' in consumption are thus necessary. The underlying 'message' must be *eat less and exercise more*! This has little to say about the rôle of '*refined-sugar*' as an important cause of obesity (*see* Table 4.1).[1]

Table 4.1:   Comparison between purchase of some dietary items between 1974 and 2016[‡*]

Fall [%] between 1974 and 2016	*Rise* [%] between 1974 and 2016
Eggs & bacon [50]	Yoghurt (500)
Meat paste sandwiches [93]	Mussels [250]
Fish and chips [66]	Take-away sandwiches [400]
Fresh peas [66]	Ready meals [1,800]

It is perhaps not surprising therefore that so much journal and newspaper space has recently been given to various theories aimed at a possible solution to the *cause* of the present *obesity crisis*. Although most attention,

‡ Figures derived from the *Office for National Statistics* – based on household food purchases.

quite correctly, has been given to diet (especially '*refined-sugar*') as well as relative inertia (lack of exercise), this chapter also focuses on several other possible causes – some resulting from the new technological age! But before tackling these problems one should perhaps again ask whether it is possible to be both healthy *and* obese, *ie,* suffer from '*benign* obesity'.

The consensus of opinion is that the two are incompatible! A study involving 60,000 individuals at the *Mount Sinai Hospital, Toronto* and published in the *Annals of Internal Medicine* confirmed that there is *no* such thing as *benign* obesity: fat people are ultimately at increased risk of heart disease and premature death. Even the fittest *obese* individuals are 30% more likely to die earlier than those of *normal* weight, according to a Swedish study involving 1.3 million men, and published in the *International Journal of Epidemlology*.[2] A minority opinion however still maintains that more research is required in this area. Some have gone even further and suggested that sooner or later, an anti-obesity 'jab' (injection) will in any case be preventive and thus solve this ongoing problem (*see* Chapter 13)![3]

Diet

The two most popular hypotheses concerning *dietary* factors and their relation to obesity involve: (i) *total* calories, and (ii) '*refined-sugar*' (sucrose) consumed in excess. The bulk of evidence is tilted towards sucrose, although other possibilities still come into the reckoning. An underlying genetic predisposition should for example be considered. So should the rôle of obese mothers – in some *via* an *epigenetic* link (*see* below).[4] Some have blamed associated hormones, alien colonic bacteria, and a minority (like the author of this book), the *fructose* moiety of sucrose. These possibilities will all be considered in this chapter.

FRUCTOSE COMPONENT OF SUCROSE

Many theories have assumed that obesity is predominantly of *dietary* origin, but simply caused by calorie *excess*. The fact that the *fructose* moiety might be responsible in its own right (*see* Chapter 8) has in my opinion received insufficient attention. The case for *fructose* as being the most important dietary constituent causing obesity is laid out in detail in that chapter.

SIMPLE CALORIE EXCESS
A straight-forward excess of dietary calories, with neglect of dietary recommendations such as that advised in the Hebrew Bible not only avoids obesity, but increases longevity![5]

EVOLUTIONARY HYPOTHESES
Sucrose, it must be recalled, consists of glucose + *fructose* – each monosaccharide being metabolised by the human body in a very different way (*see* Chapter 8), thereby creating an hypothesis that the *fructose* moiety of sucrose is the responsible culprit. Although *not* proven, the following hypothesis maintains that perhaps as much as 15 million years ago a predecessor of *Homo sapiens* (a subhuman primate – possibly a chimpanzee) possessed a gene which mutated and is subsequently inherited by present-day humans. This gene controlled *uricase,* and in order to store fat during cold spells and famines, was switched off in order to divert *fructose* (derived at that time entirely from fruit and vegetables) to adipose tissue. An excess of ingested *fructose* in present-day diets continues however to be diverted into fat and one metabolic side-product – uric acid – subsequently produces *gout*. A successor of this sub-human gene has survived in at least one of the ape's descendants – *H sapiens*. Its mutation allows *fructose* metabolism and hence uric acid (a bi-product of *fructose* metabolism), to be removed but only at too slow a rate to cope with the colossal amount of '*refined-sugar*' in the diet of modern-day primates. This hypothesis thus explains not only the current *obesity* epidemic, but also the escalation of cases of *gout* – a consequence of excessive uric acid accumulation. This is a potential answer to the *cause* of the epidemic, and once again highlights a requirement for closer co-operation between the medical and veterinary professions.[6]

Another hypothesis, based on the newly created subject of *epigenetics* (*see* below), incriminates *gluttony* in past generations. A gene with a controlling effect on obesity has had its expressiveness modified by obesity in past generations, so that resultant progeny thus has, as a result, a propensity to obesity.[7]

CONTEMPORARY GENETIC INFLUENCE

That recent genetic influences are in some way involved now seems virtually certain, although the issue has yet to be totally resolved. In a small proportion of cases, obesity is likely to be entirely under genetic control, but overall this probably only applies to a little more than *one-fifth* of cases, and no *single* gene has to date been proven responsible, a conclusion based on a study involving 340,000 individuals, and meta-analysis of 114 papers worldwide which was published in the journal *Nature*. A review of risk was also published in the *British Medical Journal* (BMJ) for 2014 indicating that consumption of an obesogenic nutrient (fried-food in this case) was indeed influenced by genetic factors; >37,000 individuals were studied, and the authors found 'at least 15 single gene forms of obesity', a mutation in a single obesity gene (MC4R) causing, for example, about one in 20 cases of *severe* childhood obesity, while the total number of obese adults with Mendelian inherited obesity was substantial. It was also concluded from that analysis that when obesity has diverse causes, different treatments should perhaps be used, *eg,* surgical management (*see* Chapter 15) in some, while lifestyle interventions are more appropriate assuming the BMI is not too high.[8]

On the supposition that obesity results from *total* calorie intake, an investigation of 2,556 pairs of twins (60% were identical) at *University College London*, and published in the journal *Obesity*, indicated that genetic factors undoubtedly convey a significant influence on BMI. At age four only 43% had a raised BMI during a time when dietary intake was regulated by their parents, but at age 10, when the children were 'given a large amount of freedom' in their choice of nutrients, this had escalated to 82%. These findings suggest that those genetically prone were *not* bound to become obese but had a propensity to do so.[9]

In another study at *King's College London*, involving 5,000 individuals (including 972 twins), published in *Nature Genetics,* and based on *total* calorie intake, a mutation in a gene coding for salivary amylase (AMY1), dated evolutionarily to introduction of agriculture, possibly as an adaptive advantage and comparable to *lactase* adaptation in milk consumption (*see* above) – an enzyme which hydrolyses starch was incriminated in the obese.[10]

AN HORMONAL THEORY

Two major appetite hormones – *leptin* and *ghrelin* – are now known to exist. It is suggested that satiety might thereby be counteracted and that an imbalance gives rise to ingestion of excess calories – causing obesity (*see* Chapter 9).

RÔLE OF COLONIC BACTERIA

This is merely also an extension of the '*refined-sugar*' (total calorie) hypothesis. '*Refined-sugar*' (sucrose) at high concentration disturbs the *milieu* within the colon (large intestine), significantly changing the composition of colonic flora. This hypothesis was developed by a geneticist at *King's College Hospital, London*, and is based on the fact that a '*refined-sugar*' (including a 'fizzy' drinks) diet alters the colonic *milieu* so that flora is changed, allowing a 'foreign' mix of bacteria to proliferate. In mice, re-institution of original colonic floral composition leads to restoration of original (thinner) body-weight. Whether this applies to *clinical* studies has however yet to be established.[11]

DIETARY *FAT* EXCESS

This hypothesis is addressed later in this chapter, and also in Chapter 12.

Other consequences of calorie reduction and 'fizzy drinks'

The fact that obesity ultimately results from an imbalance between total calorie input and output was again emphasised by a *Times* columnist in early 2015. Low-fat nutrients, advertised as containing fewer calories than full-fat ones, often contain an excess of '*refined-sugar*' and as a result calorie-value remains high. High calorie and '*refined-sugar*' content of breakfast cereals was again stressed by the *Sunday Times* in late 2014.[12] That '*refined-sugar*' and 'junk food' content is actually *increasing* in some, has also been highlighted in a recent investigation.[13]

An obsession with an *excess* of ingested calories continues and refuses to 'go away'; all other theories of causation of obesity now seem to have been largely disregarded.[14] However, in any unsolved crisis, *all* possibilities must be examined.

Results of a study involving 3,000 women, carried out by the *University of Surrey* in 2013 showed that almost 50% of *normal*-weight women apparently now feel guilty when ingesting carbohydrate in any form, recommended intake being 250g daily.[15] *'Fizzy drinks'* have been targets of the 'war on sugar', one canister of which sometimes contains at least the daily sugar allowance for an adult! In addition they contain neither fruit nor vegetables. As most British adults get an average of 11 (instead of the recommended five) per cent of energy from sugar, water and fruit should be consumed rather than a 'fizzy drink'.[16] Obsession also in young women in particular, with *'juice'* – 'juicerexia' – accompanied by a disregard for solid foods, can lead to serious ill-health; this is part of a food 'fad' – with *thinness* in mind – highlighted in an alarming report in which 'actresses, singers and reality TV stars' were apparently all involved. This is one of the anorexic lifestyles adopted by teenage girls, and constitutes a common 'eating disorder' aimed at weight-reduction. It is founded on the misapprehension that juice (which obviously lacks fibre, vitamins, etc) is devoid of calories derived from *'refined-sugar'*.[17]

Incidentally, numerous *complications*, including an association with early puberty and breast cancer in young women has been demonstrated in a US study involving 5,583 girls of 9–14 years, carried out at *Harvard Medical School* between 1996 and 2001; those who consumed 1.5 'servings of sugary drinks' daily began menstruating 2.7 months earlier than those who drank less than two sugary drinks per week, and early puberty is a proven risk factor for breast cancer. Another article indicated that teenage brains and hence memory can be damaged by 'sugary drinks'.[18] Although these findings, published in *Hippocampus*, were carried out in rats, researchers at *Southern California University* saw no reason why they could not be extrapolated to *H sapiens*. 'Fizzy drinks' can also be associated with flabbiness around the waist, as shown in a study of 749 people over age five carried out over ten years at the *Texas Health Center* at *San Antonio*, and published in the *Journal of the American Geriatrics Society*; this showed an increase in waist measurement which directly correlated with numbers of 'fizzy drinks' consumed; however, whether this resulted from *'refined-sugar'* or artificial sweeteners was apparently unclear.[19]

Cost of junk-food

Healthy food is more *expensive* (and becoming increasingly so) compared with 'junk' food, and confirmed by a study at the *University of Cambridge* and published in *Plos One*. There were 50% more kebab, pizza and fried chicken outlets in Norfolk in 2015 than was the case in 1997, the greatest increase being in 'deprived areas'. Rich and poor are affected, and hence probably too much blame has been apportioned to individuals themselves. This finding could be 'fuelling the obesity crisis'. *Lifestyle* is also important, according to findings of a study involving 8,314 people at the *University of New York*; those who eat at their desk (*see also* Chapter 13) are, for example, more likely to be obese, and have low vitamin and higher LDL cholesterol concentrations.[20]

ALCOHOL

Increased *alcohol* consumption, together with an excess of '*refined-sugar*' as a substitute for 'proper' meals, has been incriminated as an 'environmental' *cause* of obesity, most evidence relating to excessive *beer* consumption – frequently associated with a 'beer belly'. A suspicion that British women drink an excess of wine (usually in evenings) compared with their French counterparts, and rarely cook with butter has also been blamed as a contributory factor to the high prevalence of obesity in Britain. French women are apparently *rarely* obese![21]

Other Views

Not all agree that the major *cause* of obesity is to be found in 'junk food and 'fizzy drinks' or that all other possibilities must be urgently considered. This theory is certainly *not* accepted by the food industry, and a recent article in the London *Times* newspaper – based on a USA study – took a very sceptical view.[22] Perhaps other dietary items are implicated. Reasoning was further confused when recommendations changed from '*refined-sugar*' to fat (*see* below). *Many* are thus biased in their opinion(s). A bizarre approach, often held by those who support the hormonal theory, is that a sweet-tasting diet drink suppresses desire to consume sweet food, and is thus superior to water![23]

Research in *rhesus monkeys* at the *University of Wisconsin–Madison* and published in *Nature Communications* has indicated that a low-calorie

(30% below normal) diet both delays ageing (*see also* Chapter 5), and also conveys a propensity to avoid *diabetes mellitus*, cardiac disease and certain malignancies – underlying mechanisms are however unclear.[24]

Why has obesity become increasingly common over the last few decades?
Many factors have been incriminated in the enormous rise in prevalence of obesity throughout the world in recent years (*see* Chapter 1), much *recent* research being focused controversially on appetite-associated hormones (*see* Chapter 9).

John Yudkin, although much of his evidence was not scientifically acceptable, rightly referred to the huge increase in production and consumption of '*refined-sugar*' ('sucrose') in the last two – *eighteenth* and *nineteenth* (*see* Prologue and Chapter 6) – centuries; during the last there was an overall 25-fold increase in world production: whereas in 1800 this was 0.25 million tonnes, in 1982 it had soared to 101 million. As he stressed, this varied enormously from country to country, and only in the last few years have 'third world' populations begun catching up! Similarly, average *individual* '*refined-sugar*' consumption has escalated: in the UK; two hundred years ago average consumption was approximately 2 kg per year, but by the mid-*nineteenth* century this had risen to 25 lbs (11 kg), and in the 1980s to 100 (45 kg). In Germany corresponding figures are 2 kg for 1825, and 36 in 1980. Much increase has been in manufactured foods, *ie,* by surreptitiously added '*refined-sugar*' to dietary constituents. A significant proportion has been targeted at infants and children (*see* Chapter 3), and as weaning has on average taken place at an earlier age, sweet foods have been introduced earlier. Also, 'fizzy' drinks, ice-cream, and chocolates (most containing added '*refined-sugar*'), have increasingly been introduced into childhood diets. As Yudkin narrated, when he was a boy, thirst was quenched with a glass of water, but when he wrote his book (in the 1960s) this requirement was solved with a glass of 'sugar-laden *cola* or [another sugar-containing] drink'. Also, by ingesting '*refined-sugar*' *between* meals the amount consumed *with* meals was substantially reduced. What is abundantly clear is that much of this increase involves 'industrial sugar', a large part of the attraction being in *presentation* of sophisticated eating and drinking products, and also in 'advances' in *advertising*-promoted sales.[25]

Does dietary fat play a part in the obesity epidemic?

As several writers, including Nina Teicholz and Matt Ridley of the *Times*, have concluded, a flawed hypothesis indicating that ingestion of excessive amounts of *saturated fat* has been the *cause* of disorders ranging from obesity to arterial disease has misled millions of individuals and organisations, including members of the *American Heart Association* over the last few decades. Ancel Keys (1906–2004), an American 'scientist', convinced a naive audience in the 1950s and 60s that ingestion of fatty foodstuffs was a major killer; this was closely allied to his later 'high blood *cholesterol*' hypothesis. Both conclusions were based largely on the fact that fat and cholesterol were both present in diseased arteries, most obvious in overweight individuals. Keys' studies are now regarded to have been based on spurious evidence, while serious flaws in his arguments were ignored. Now, evidence has shown that *dietary* fat is *not* in itself harmful, and furthermore does *not* cause obesity. As an example, the 'Atkins diet' – formulated by an American cardiologist Robert Coleman Atkins (1930–2003) – which contains a great deal of fat – *lowers* weight more effectively and rapidly than one containing an excess of sucrose and little fat! This change in thought has been corroborated by a member of the British medical profession! The hypothesis that *saturated fat* is associated with obesity is perhaps the reverse of the case, and has also been confirmed in several well-conducted clinical trials.[26] This has added further evidence that the main dietary culprit in obesity lies in '*refined-sugar*' rather than fat. Not all agree, however, that *complete* exoneration of dietary fat is correct; the fat hypothesis in fact still has some supporters.[27]

Ethnic Factors

In 2012 'white Britons' were shown to be twice more likely than those with a black or Asian background to suffer from a 'limiting long-standing illness' such as: hypertension, cardiac abnormality or bronchial asthma, all being complications worsened by obesity. The cause of these differences, derived from records at the *Office for National Statistics* were possibly the result of an unsatisfactory diet in white families (*see* above), coupled with higher levels of alcohol consumption. But obesity can affect any ethnic group; after all we are of the same species – *H sapiens* – and *all* originally even shared an identical skin colour![28]

Other Factors Influencing Obesity

Impact of *social class* is complex; perceived differences in how obesity is viewed also enter this arena. Total energy consumption varies in different regions and countries, and most societies are becoming increasingly reliant on energy-dense, large-portioned, fast-food meals; while this already applies to most 'westernised' populations, it is increasingly relevant in the 'third world'. The price of *processed* food has declined compared with that of fruit and vegetables, which in consequence are being eaten less often. A diet containing both less sugar and fat, together with increased *physical activity* (*see* below) are crucial in the *war against obesity*, while anti-obesity drugs might eventually contribute in some cases. Surgical techniques designed to reduce gastric volume, and/or small-intestinal length, are occasionally necessary in a severe case (*see* Chapter 15).[29]

Physical activity (*see also* Chapter 12)

Balanced against over-consumption of a dietary item – arguably '*refined-sugar*' (sucrose) – are increased levels of *physical activity* which have currently plummeted. 'On average, every individual consumes 25 calories in excess of that which he/she expends daily; although this does not seem much … it accumulates over the years, and thus makes us fat'. Ten thousand school playing fields were sold off between 1979 and 1997 (Britain's Prime Minister between 1979 and 1990 was the Conservative, Margaret Thatcher), and furthermore 'nearly one in 10 adults does not presently walk continuously for even five minutes daily. Among suggested solutions are: (i) banning cars once a week, and (ii) providing more sports facilities at the workplace, accompanied by more time to use them.[30]

Several articles have emphasised that a sedentary existence is probably a major cause in the *obesity explosion*. Children under 18 years from Scotland are for example, *seriously* lacking in physical activity, and those from England are not far behind (*see* Chapter 3). A survey which included: the USA, Nigeria, Mexico, and Australia, carried out in 15 countries and published in the *Journal of Physical Activity and Health* concluded that children in Scotland, owing to 'temptations of [modern] technology' are in the lowest grade, being lower than Mozambique and New Zealand. A majority of Scottish boys watch television and/or play computer games for more than four hours daily. There is hope that a new game – 'Pokémon Go' – will take obese children 'out of the house' and as a result encourage increased exercise; but perhaps it is too early to be enthusiastic! In addition, only one in seven ate more than five portions of fruit and vegetables daily, while average sugar and fat intake was in both cases higher than recommended.[31]

Other 'avoidable' causes of obesity
OBESE MOTHERS

Realisation that obesity sometimes begins *before* birth (*see above* and Chapter 3) was not appreciated, and published until 2015; since then, several papers have alluded to this fact. Fifty per cent of pregnant women are now known to be either overweight or obese according to British hospital records of 36,000 women attending 80 hospitals. The problem in Britain is worse in the north country, although in the London area, 36% were declared overweight. This study concluded that *all* women should be of normal weight and fitness *before* pregnancy to avoid having obese babies, abortions, stillbirths, miscarriages or difficult labours. Women are advised however *not* to attempt weight-reduction *during* pregnancy. In Scotland advice is more severe, obese women being told *not* to become pregnant until their weight is normal.[32]

Another study, at *New York University* and published in *Science Translational Medicine* asserted that *Caesarean sections* increase risk of both obesity and diabetes in the mother. This might be associated with altered colonic bacterial flora arising from associated broad-spectrum antibiotic therapy! The increased rate of Caesarean-section – especially in America – is thus the source of considerable concern.' Infant-feeding with artificial, as opposed to breast-milk, has also been associated with obesity; the authors considered that development of the immune system might explain these findings![33]

EPIGENETIC FACTORS

It is clear that some overweight women give birth to babies who, judging by their telomeres are significantly older than predicted, but when several generations are heavier than they should be it is possible that *epigenetics* is entering the scenario (*see* above). Epigenetics is essentially an extension or reinvention of Lamarckism, the basic theory surrounding the *gene* being fundamentally unaltered, but it is now clear that the gene 'does not have all its own way'; it can be inactivated by events from the past (*ie,* the lifestyle of his/her ancestors). In fact the role of DNA is less rigid than the Darwin-Wallace theory allows; genes can in fact be turned 'on and off'! Also on this theme, Mukherjee has described the Dutch famine of 1944–5 following which *obesity* and cardiac disease were more common in the next *two* generations (this might have been related to a specific (*eg,* a vitamin) deficiency during pregnancy, but the actual cause has not been established, and it might be part of a strategy for survival. *Epigenetics* in fact *regulates gene expression* (*see* above), and genetic influence in response to environmental (including availability of food) factors. The body is thus in effect reprogrammed for survival.[34]

OTHER SUGGESTED CAUSES
Many of these factors are dealt with elsewhere in the book. Emphasis has concentrated on colonic and cerebral (including *stress*) factors and sleep deficit. A study in mice, and published in *Cell Reports* has suggested that obesity in a woman's parents or grandparents might be 'inherited' and is thus a factor operating *before* pregnancy (possibly a further example of *epigenetics – see* above) – causing obesity before conception. Should this be confirmed in *H sapiens* it might be significant because childrens' diets also tend to mirror those of their parents.

Conclusion
The *cause(s)* of obesity is certainly multi-factorial. Evolution and genetics clearly play a part. While an unsatisfactory diet (*'refined-sugar'* being primarily incriminated) and exercise deficiency are obviously important, other possibilities, in particular obese mothers and epigenetics, have also entered the scenario. In this author's opinion, the rôle of *fructose* has been seriously underplayed in this controversy. Not all agree that a dietary factor (probably *'refined-sugar'*) is the *major* culprit – most *sceptics* either being associated with the food industry, or are members of the British government.

Reference and notes

1 T Whipple. Secret of long life is 1,500 calories a day. *Times, Lond* 2017; January 18: 5; P Willan. Weight gain. *Ibid* 2017; January 2: 24; T Whipple. Why healthier eating is making us fatter. *Ibid* 2016; December 31: 31.

2 G Taubes. The science of obesity: what do we really know about what makes us fat? *Br med J* 2013: 346 (April 20): 16–19; G Taubes. *The Case Against Sugar* London: Portobello Books 2016: 365; O Moody. Half of overweight people are healthy, scientists admit. *Times, Lond* 2016; February 5: 23; T Whipple. Obese but healthy? It's a big, fat myth. *Ibid* 2013: December 3: 10; C Smyth. It's just a load of porkies: there's no such thing as fat and fit. *Ibid* 2015; December 21: 9. (*See also*: Z Morris. The 10 rules for staying lean for life. *Times 2, Lond* 2015: January 10: 9; A Ellson. Teething problems at Amazon's new grocer service. *Times, Lond* 2016; June 8: 39; A Ellson. Online shops need to take the rap for too much waste. *Ibid* 2016; June 18: 30; K Gibbons. Doctors should prescribe nuts and greens. *Ibid* 2016; July 22: 4; A Malhotra. Nuts, olive oil and vegetables are the best heart medicine. *Ibid* 2016; July 22: 30.)

3 O Moody. Injection could help to burn away the fat. *Ibid* 2016; July 1: 24.

4 H Devlin. Genetic key to childhood obesity. *Ibid* 2014; 24 April: 17. (*See also*: O Moody. Don't blame fat people for obesity, says weight tsar. *Ibid* 2016; April 8: 1, 4; T Whipple. Harm from a poor diet felt for generations. *Ibid* 2016; June 17: 12; C Smyth. Half of today's mothers-to-be are overweight. *Ibid* 2016; March 3: 23.)

5 Op cit. See note 1 above; H Devlin. Fewer calories for longer life. *Ibid* 2014; April 2: 13; G Sandeman. Adults should cut calories to 1,800 per day. *Ibid* 2017; December 27: 2. Anonymous. The good Cookbook: following the Daniel diet, how else could the Bible inspire weight loss? *Ibid* 2013; November 29: 32; (*See also*: K Lay. Poor diets are blamed for more early deaths than smoking. *Ibid* 2015; September 15: 19; G Ridsdale. Biblical diets. *Ibid* November 31: 27.)

6 J Leake. Obesity epidemic linked to chubby chimp gene. *Sunday Times, Lond* 2015; November 15: 27.

7   A Klein. Obesity is passed on down generations. *New Scientist* 2016; July 23: 10; S Mukherjee. *The Gene – an intimate history*. London: Bodley Head 2016: 393–410 (*See also*: A Malhotra. Nuts, olive oil and vegetables are the best heart medicine. *Times, Lond* 2016; July 22: 30; *G C Cook. The Milk Enzyme: adventures with the human* lactase *polymorphism*. Ely, Cambridgeshire: Melrose Books 2016: 118.)

8   Op cit. *See* note 4 (Devlin) above; O Moody, K Lay. Obesity is in the genes for millions of people. *Times, Lond* 2015: February 12: 4; A I F Blakemore, J L Buxton. Obesity, genetic risk, and environment: genetic makeup can inflate effects of bad diet. *Br med J* 2014 (March 22); 348: 7; T Whipple. 'Atkins gene' reveals why obesity can run in the family. *Times, Lond* 2014; March 31: 1–2; K M Livingstone, C Celis-Morales, G D Papandonatos *et al*. FTO genotype and weight loss. *Br med J* 2016 (September 24); 354: 4707.

9   *Ibid.*

10   *Ibid.*

11   J Leake. Fast food kills bugs that keep you thin. *Sunday Times, Lond* 2015; May 10: 10. (*See also*: T Whipple. Junk food kills bugs that fight illness. *Times, Lond* 2015; May 11: 4; O Moody. Western diet destroys healthy bacteria. *Ibid* 2015; June 4: 14; O Moody. Bacteria found in thin people could help to fight obesity. *Ibid* 2015; June 15: 20; J Russell. Counting the calories won't make you thin: evidence is growing that the destruction of our gut bacteria by processed food is the real enemy. *Ibid* 2016: February 18: 26; P Bee. Gut instinct: Do you have the right bacteria? it's the new A-list craze that claims the secret to weight loss lies in your stomach. *Times 2, Lond* 2015; July 28: 6–7; T Spector. *The Diet Myth*. London: Weidenfield and Nicolson: 2016; K Lay. Athlete's gut bacteria could help you get the fitness bug. *Times, Lond* 2012; August 21: 19.)

12   D Aaronovitch. Forget the faddy diets and go back to basics: the debate over fat and carbs obscures the truth that consuming fewer calories than we burn is the only way to slim. *Ibid* 2015; February 12: 25; G Sandeman. Adults should cut calories to 1,800 per day. *Ibid* 2017; December 27: 2.

13   C Smyth, K Lay. Fat chance of beating obesity as takeaways rise by

50%. *Ibid* 2015; April 2: 38.

14 Anonymous. We must eat less. *Ibid* 2017; February 17: 28; K Greenhalgh. Mr Micawber's rule. *Ibid* 2016; May 21: 21; O Wright. Bad figures hid truth on how Britain is overeating. *Ibid* 2016; August 8: 13.

15 A Thomson. We've got to stop eating ourselves to death: shaming doesn't work. A combination of sugar tax and clever incentives to reduce intake of bad food is the answer. *Ibid* 2015: December 2: 33; K Lay. Sugary drinks are blamed for 184,000 deaths every year. *Ibid* 2015; June 30: 12; O Moody. Beware the calories in low-fat foods. *Ibid* 2014; May 30: 16; H Devlin. Nearly half of women suffer 'carb guilt'. *Ibid* 2013; December 30: 14.

16 O Moody. Junk foods not to blame for obesity crisis, scientists say. *Ibid* 2015; November 6: 27.

17 P Ellis. Sugar-packed cereals making us fat. *Sunday Times, Lond* 2015; December 14: 34; K Gibbons. Give breakfast a miss if you want to lose weight. *Times, Lond* 2016; March 25: 11; K Lay. Breakfast cereal as sugary as seven chocolate biscuits. *Ibid* 2015; January 28: 24; M Mosley. Crash diets, juicing and exercise: 10 myths about weight loss: is breakfast essential if you're trying to lose weight? Is it really better to eat little and often? *Times 2, Lond* 2014; June 14: 6–7; Anonymous. Lunch 'loaded with sugar' at attractions. *Times, Lond* 2016; October 19: 4.

18 K Lay. Fizzy drinks linked to early puberty and breast cancer. *Ibid* 2015; January 28: 24; Anonymous. Sugary drinks can damage teenage brains. *Ibid* 2014; October 9: 25.

19 C Smyth. Fizzy drinks are target in new war on sugar. *Ibid* 2014; June 27: 1, 2. (*See also*: H Rumbelow. Dinner through a straw could spell juicerexia. *Times 2, Lond* 2014; May 26: 6–7.)

20 K Lay. Junk food gets more attractive as cost of healthy eating soars. *Times, Lond* 2014; October 9: 25.

21 K Lay. Diet drinks put inches on your waist. *Ibid* 2015: March 17: 24; K Gibbons. Wine-loving British women 'are too fat'. *Ibid* 2014; February 4: 8; K Gibbons. Middle aged in denial over alcohol and weight. *Ibid* 2016; December 28: 1, 4.

22 A Boyd. Don't blame sugar. *Ibid* 2015; September 7: 32; O Moody.

Junk foods not to blame for obesity crisis, scientists say. *Ibid* November 6: 27; E Roberts. Sugar rush. *Ibid* 2014; January 28: 29; G Jones. Sugar. *Ibid 2014;* January 14: 27; Anonymous. Sweet diet drinks 'better than water' to help you lose weight. *Ibid* November 11: 11.

23 S Hazel. Why sweet and fatty foods make us keep eating. *Ibid* 2016; July 13: 14.

24 H Devlin. Fewer calories for longer life. *Ibid* 2014; April 2: 13.

25 J Yudkin. *Pure, white and deadly: how sugar is killing us and what we can do to stop it.* London: Penguin Books 2012: 200; K Lay. Diet drinks put inches on your waist. *Times, Lond* 2015; March 17: 24.; A Shanahan. Man v Fat. *Times 2, Lond* 2015; January 5: 2–3, January 6: 4–5; February 4: 8; T Whipple. Why fat people have a better nose for food. *Times, Lond* 2015: July 8: 25; J Boswell, E Griffiths. Restaurants' savoury dishes pile on sugar. *Sunday Times, Lond* 2016; March 6: 17; K Lay. Poor diets are blamed for more early deaths than smoking. *Times, Lond* 2015; September 15: 19.

26 N Teicholz. *The Big Fat Surprise.* London: Scribe 2015: 369; Anonymous. Professor Michael Oliver. *Ibid* 2015: July 10: 56; C Smyth. Don't worry about butter, bread is the real problem. *Ibid* 2016; June 30: 20; K Gibbons. Butter is good but olive oil is better. *Ibid* 2016; July 6: 25; M Ridley. More eggs, please. Cholesterol is OK now. *Ibid* 2015: May 25: 23; D Kromhout. Where the latest US dietary guidelines are heading: so farewell dietary cholesterol and total fat as risk factors worth worrying about. *Br med J* 2015; 351 (August 18): 5;

27 O Moody. Professor who backed butter now says it's best avoided. *Times, Lond* 2016; July 20: 15. (*See also*: H Devlin. Too much cheese and meat in your middle age is a recipe for early death. *Ibid* 2014; March 5: 4.)

28 K Gibbons. Britain 'lags behind US in obesity fight.' *Ibid* 2014; January 8: 19; R Blakely. Fat Americans urged to diet and save the planet. *Ibid* 2015; February 23: 34; B Wilson. *First Bite: how we learn to eat.* London: Fourth Estate 2016: 126; (*See also* ref 7 (Cook) above.)

29 C Smyth. Children going hungry in 'Oliver Twist Britain'. *Times,*

Lond 2014; May 2: 25; K Gibbons. Affluent girls are more likely to become obese than boys. *Ibid* 2016; October 11: 1.

30 A Radnor, R Gledhill. Bursts of exercise 'key to weight loss'. *Ibid* 2013; December 3: 10; P Bee. Power steps: why walking is the best exercise at any age. *Times 2, Lond* 2014; August 23: 4–5; N Woolcock. Live longer with vigorous exercise, middle-aged told. *Times, Lond* 2015; April 7: 20; O Moody. Want to live longer? Take a short stroll round the office. *Ibid* 2015; May 1: 8; A Thomson. Pokémon Go shows the route to healthy profit: the gaming craze is getting obese children off the sofa and should encourage the PM to stand up to the sugar lobby. *Ibid* 2016; July 20: 25.

31 K Lay. One in three people is a couch potato. *Ibid* 2017; April 3: 10 N Woolcock. Live longer with vigorous exercise, middle-aged told. *Ibid* 2015; April 7: 20; Anonymous. Walk for 15 minutes a day to cut risk of an early death. *Ibid* 2016; June 15: 22; L Bannerman. Beer, dry bread and manly exercise: keeping fit the 1830s way. *Ibid* 2016; December 30: 3.

32 M Wade. Don't have babies, health chief tells addicts and obese. *Ibid* 2016: May 27: 6; C Smyth. Half of today's mothers-to-be are over-weight. *Ibid* 2016; March 3: 23; Anonymous. Unhealthy diet during pregnancy raises rise of ADHD. *Ibid* 2016; August 19: 18; M Porter. The fight against obesity begins in the womb. *Times 2, Lond* 2015; July 21: 6; S-K Templeton. Ops for women to prevent fat babies. *Sunday Times, Lond* 2015; July 19: 18 S-K Templeton. Obese mothers strain maternity units. *Ibid* 2017; December 17: 4.

33 O Moody. Caesarean deliveries increase risk of obesity and diabetes. *Ibid* 2016; June 16: 21; C Smyth. C-section babies face raised obesity risk. *Ibid* 2016; September 7: 1,4.

34 T Whipple. Harm from a poor diet felt for generations. *Ibid* 2016; June 17: 12; K Amey. Epigenetics: your lifestyle can change your genes. *New Scientist* 2015; December 12: 39; O Moody. Obese mothers can pass faulty DNA to babies. *Times, Lond* 2014; February 11: 6; C Smyth. Babies of obese mothers born 'older'. *Ibid* 2016; October 18: 10.

CHAPTER 5:

The quest for sweetness: a 'sweet tooth' and the historical attraction to honey

Why were humans so desirous of sweetness – be it '*refined*-sugar' or another sweet tasting substance? The origin of *Homo sapiens*' 'sweet tooth' is of course lost in time! However, the quest for sweetness has been splendidly outlined in a book by food anthropologist Sidney Mintz (1922–2015): *Sweetness and power: the place of sugar in modern history* (1985).[1]

The first substance, apart from fruit, to be attractive to *H sapiens* on account of its *sweet taste* was naturally-occurring honey. Exactly when that was is of course again impossible to discover. Mankind, especially when young, has always had a craving for sweet foods. Honey has thus been used as a specific sweetener for countless millennia. As John Yudkin has emphasised, until about 2,500 years ago, satiety was obtained from fruit and honey (*see* below). During the *seventeenth* and *eighteenth* centuries, however, honey was slowly replaced by cane-sugar, initially not well-refined. This chapter dwells on honey before the transition to '*refined-sugar*'– which is now proving both disastrous for modern humans, but constitutes a major source of income for the *sugar industry* which is addressed in Chapter 6.

The existence of sweetness in early *H sapiens* is no better exemplified than by an *idealistic* 'vision' set out in the account given in the book of *Exodus* in the Hebrew Bible and Torah:

A LAND OF MILK AND **HONEY**

There is a great deal of controversy as to exactly what this text means! Honey might of course be a reference to *nectar* in fruit rather than bees' honey, while milk only flows when there are verdant pastures upon which livestock can feed. Overall, the phrase probably relates to an idealised fertile and *sweet* 'Promised Land' (*ie, ancient* Israel). Sweetness (derived at that time from honey) was therefore a goal to be sought above all others (and was coupled with animals' *milk* – another commodity – in an *idealised* environment).[2] Several other references in the Old and New Testaments refer to both honey and manna – most obtained from southern Arabia (present-day Yemen and Oman). The *Seamen's Hospital Society* (SHS)'s *Quarterly Magazine* for example, contains this reference to honey in southern Arabia:

> [commenting on a gift of Hadhramaut honey to the SHS from the Secretary of State for the Colonies, it recorded: This] honey was a gift from a Sultan of the Aden Protectorate who visited London for the [1937] Coronation; it has a much stronger flavour than … English honey and is of [a] darker colour. It is … a delicacy in southern Arabia and has been thought … to be the manna mentioned in the Bible.[3]

Honey in recent history

Farmers were apparently using both honey and beeswax at the dawn of British agriculture, while stone-age or paleolithic[§] communities were '[removing] honey from beehives 9,000 years ago'.[4] Furthermore, there is evidence assembled by investigators at the University of Bristol and published in the journal *Nature*, that honey taken from beehives was present in a neolithic town founded in about 7,200 BC in eastern Anatolia.[5]

Before enthusiasm for '*refined-sugar*' (sucrose) arose, sweetness was thus provided by honey; this probably began when *H sapiens* became domesticated, and later when agriculture had become widespread by the first century and, at a time when the Roman poet Virgil (70BC–19BC) clearly described beekeeping. Beekeepers originally had their own saints, and honey was of course prominent in two developing monotheistic religions during the first millennium AD – Christianity and Islam; it was used in *Christianity* to sweeten both food and medicines, but its fermentation produced mead – exploited by monasteries and other religious organisations; beeswax candles were also used in *Christian* liturgies. In *Islam*, alcohol was strictly forbidden from the founding of that religion, but honey was commended in the Koran both as a *sweetener*

---

§ The *paleolithic* period dated from about 2.6 million to 10,000 years BC. This era was followed by the *mesolithic*.

in tea, and also for its medicinal properties, the originator of the faith – the Prophet Mohammed – recommended honey for its healing properties and use in mint tea – sweetened by this commodity – which is of course freely allowed. Honey has remained an important sweetener in the Middle East – much being imported from both Pakistan and the USA.

Sweetness in 2017
Popularity of honey has risen markedly in recent years; in 2005, for example, sales overtook those of marmalade, and in 2013 in Britain totalled £112 million, compared with £119 million spent on jams and conserves. Increased use has not been solely for its *sweetness* properties (*see* below). Another article indicates that for the first time, sales of honey had overtaken those of jam in Waitrose stores.[6] So great has been the recent quest for honey, that demand is outstripping rates of production, and in fact more jars of *manuka* honey are being sold than actually produced! Between 2,000 and 3,000 tonnes of manuka honey were produced in New Zealand, and it is now being marketed around the world under that name.[7] The makers of 'Sugar Puffs' have in fact re-named their product *'Honey Monster Puffs'*, increase in the *honey* component apparently being accompanied by a reduction in *'refined-sugar'*.[8]

It has been asked: Is this rise in popularity of honey justified? As a replacement for *'refined-sugar'*, the answer is undoubtedly in the affirmative, but as for other uses, including antimicrobial properties (*see* below) the answer is far less clear. Manuka honey (*see* above) is undoubtedly a good antimicrobial agent, but other honey products (some poor substitutes) less so.[9]

The bee population
Slowly, as research published in the journal *Plos One* indicates, we are beginning to gain an insight into the intimate life of honey bees.[10] There have been numerous recent warnings that populations of bees (and hence honey supplies) are in serious decline, possibly resulting from overuse of *neonicotinoid* pesticides – connected with new techniques for delivering pesticides to crops, which incidentally include strawberries and apples. However, some observers, including Matt Ridley, a *Times* columnist, consider that this alarm is misplaced and that bees are actually thriving![11]

HAZARDS FACED BY HONEY-COLLECTORS
Although beekeeping seems an attractive hobby or occupation, it is of paramount importance that pitfalls are avoided, for being stung by a bee, although an unusual experience, can be extremely painful.[12] Also, dangers faced by collectors of honey in Bengal, India, have recently been outlined; in a *Times* article, it was estimated that by the end of the wild honey collecting season, death toll from tigers 'could be 20 or more'. Other dangers come from snakes, sharks and crocodiles. Bee stings are therefore of only minor importance.[13]

Alternative uses for honey
Historically, honey has been used in wound-healing. The fact that some types of honey (notably manuka) have proven antimicrobial properties is now well known (*see* above) and with increasing antibiotic-resistance in bacteria, it is likely that more will be heard of this in the future.[14]

The transition to refined-sugar (sucrose)
Movement *away* from honey as a *sweetener* has occurred over three or four centuries (*see* Chapter 6). Although the value of '*refined-sugar*' in sweetening food and drink has proved over this period to be highly satisfactory, its ingestion is of course accompanied by serious side-effects which this book is attempting to enumerate!

The *World Health Organisation* (WHO) recommendation for '*refined-sugar*' restriction is currently for a maximum of *five* teaspoons daily. In company with almost every foodstuff or drink widely consumed by *H sapiens*, '*refined-sugar*' or sucrose has (unlike honey) numerous *serious* side-effects (*see* Chapter 11). Although known for many decades that it is largely responsible for dental caries, systemic problems – especially prevalence of *type-2- diabetes mellitus* – have perhaps not been so widely appreciated. Who would suspect, for example, that tomato soup or a tin of baked beans is loaded with the 'sweet stuff'?

Longevity and honey
Unlike honey, '*refined-sugar*' has a reverse effect on *longevity*. Honey has long been associated (correctly or incorrectly) with prolongation of life, several examples being:

- Thomas Carn who died on January 28 1588 at the age of 207; this is corroborated by the Parish Register at St Leonard's Church, Shoreditch,
- Thomas Parr who died on November 16 1635 at the age of 152,
- Henry Jenkins who died at 169 years on December 8 1670,
- Catherine, Countess of Desmond who died at 148 years in 1612, and
- Thomas Damme reached 154.

Other examples are of people who lived until: 185, 170, 152, 150, 145, 143, 140, 137, 136, 130, 124, and 104 years. There are also numerous older examples. Although these are all from the *seventeenth* or *eighteenth* centuries or before, when documentation was far less accurate than today, it is undoubtedly true that *all* achieved unusual longevity! The role of associated under-nutrition cannot, of course, be evaluated.

An investigation on *rhesus* monkeys (*Macaca mulatta*), and published in *Nature Communications*, might be relevant in this context. This indicated that a low-calorie diet, lacking sucrose (and approximately 30% lower in calories than the normal diet) both delayed the ageing process and also extended life-span; furthermore, incidence of diabetes mellitus, cardiac disease and 'some cancers' – all associated with obesity – were reduced. Theories accounting for this finding are that:

- when food is scarce, increased resources, in terms of calories, are directed at tissue maintenance – resulting in a protective effect, and
- fasting is associated with production of proteins, which are protective of cells in facing oxidative stress – which in turn counteracts ageing and its complications.

Whether or not this finding (clearly exacerbated by a 'sweet tooth') is applicable to *H sapiens* remains at present unknown.[15]

Conclusion
Until introduction of '*refined-sugar*' (sucrose) as the principal sweetener (*see* Chapter 6), naturally occurring honey was a major component of

the human diet. This was virtually free from side-effects and associated, rightly or wrongly, with increased longevity.

Although some evidence exists that honey consumption in 2017 is increasing, with a rapidly increasing population demand this will inevitably exceed supply. Thus, for the foreseeable future, '*refined-sugar*' will predominate.

References and notes

1   Anonymous. Sidney Mintz: food anthropologist who traced the origins of Britain's love of sugar. *Times, Lond* 2016; January 5: 54.
2   Holy Bible. *Exodus* 3: 8; O Moody. Stone Age settlers had a taste for honey. *Ibid* 2015: November 12: 33.
3   G C Cook. *Origin of a medical specialty: the Seamen's Hospital Society and tropical medicine.* St Albans: Tropzam 2012: 58.
4   Op cit. *See* note 1 above.
5   O Moody. Rise of the healthy breakfast gives shoppers a taste for honey. *Times, Lond* 2014; March 15: 16.
6   O Moody. Jam is overtaken by healthy honey. *Ibid* 2014: October 22: 17.
7   Anonymous. Sales of 'superfood' honey push bees past limit. *Ibid* 2015; May 4: 18; T Whipple. Test to stamp out honey laundering. *Ibid* 2017; January 24: 17; J Leake. Bee careful: that £45 honey may be fake. *Sunday Times, Lond* 2017; February 5: 3.
8   G Swerling. Tell 'em about the honey (but not the sugar). *Times, Lond* 2014; October 18: 19.
9   L Slater. Is honey as healthy as we think it is? As sales of honey soar in the supermarkets [it should be asked] whether it really is good for us. *Times 2, Lond* 2014; November 15: 8.
10 L Holden. Pooh joins fight to save the honey bee. *Times, Lond* 2015; June 25: 23; T Whipple. Flight of bumblebee suggests they have unique personalities. *Ibid* 2016; August 5: 11; J Leake. New crop protection is the bees' knees. *Sunday Times, Lond* 2015; November 15: 25; Anonymous. The bee's knees. *Times, Lond* 2017; August 16: 4. (*See also*: N Badshah. New bee is creating a buzz. *Ibid* 2016; October 17: 12; D Goulson. *Bee Quest.* London; Jonathan Cape 2016: 233; Anonymous. The plight of the bumblebee: several species are under threat. *Times, Lond* 2017; January 28: 81; G Narwan. Sweet solution takes the sting out of bees' fight for survival. *Ibid* 2017; February 9: 14; M Bridge. Drone bee swarms to fertilise flowers. *Ibid* 2017; February 10: 19; B Webster. Bees benefit from cuts to mowing. *Ibid* 2017: April 6: 13; T Whipple. Bees learn football with the help of a sweet goal. *Ibid* 2017; February 24: 24; B Hoyle. Beekeeper stung by theft of 488 hives. *Ibid* 2017; January 28: 43; Anonymous. Queen's

beekeeper dosed hives with banned drug. *Ibid* 2017; January 19: 21.)

11 T Whipple. Pesticides 'make male bees sterile'. *Ibid* 2016: July 27: 10; Anonymous. Plan Bee: pesticides which harm bees have no place in modern farming. *Ibid* 2016; August 17: 27; B Webster. Pesticides blamed for dramatic decline in number of wild bees. *Ibid* 2016; August 17: 9; B Webster. Arrival of alien hornet poses threat to bees. *Ibid* 2016; September 21: 3; B Webster. 'Bee-harming' pesticides face total ban. *Ibid* 2017; March 24: 15; B Webster. Pesticide firms reject their own study's findings of harm to bees. *Ibid* 2017; June 30: 19; M Ridley. Don't weep for the sad decline of bees. They're thriving. *Ibid* 2015; May 15: 30; M Ridley. Gove's ban on neonicotinoids will harm insects. *Ibid* 2017; November 10: 30. (*See also*: J Leake. Survival of bumblebees under threat from farm pesticides. *Sunday Times, Lond* 2017; August 27:7.)

12 H Prevett. Where work is a hive of activity and mistakes really hurt. *Times, Lond* 2016; March 31: 45; D Waller. Bees are a sticky business but life is sweet. *Ibid* 2017; August 31: 47.

13 R Pagnamenta. The most dangerous job in the world? Honey collectors face deadly foe to put food on table. *Ibid* 2015; April 18: 43.

14 G C Cook. *Before the 'Germ Theory': a history of cause and management of infectious disease before 1900.* Ely, Cambridgeshire: Melrose Books 2015: 202; M Haynes. Sweet solution. *Times, Lond* 2015; April 3: 36; K Gibbons. Honey offers a sweeter way to stop infections spreading. *Ibid* 2016; September 27: 23; W M Sheard. Honey trap. *Ibid* 2016; September 29: 30; M Badger. Honey to bridle at. *Ibid* 2016; September 30: 32.

15 H Devlin. Fewer calories for longer life. *Ibid* 2014; April 2: 13. (*See also*: Anonymous. On this day: we must eat less. *Ibid* 2017; February 17: 28; K Lay, R Bennett. Living to 90 will be the new norm. *Ibid* 2017; February 22: 9.)

CHAPTER 6:

The transition from honey to *'refined-sugar'*

This book is largely devoted to the side-effects of a natural product which succeeded honey several centuries ago. Therefore, before giving details of the transition, a few pages on the origin of this toxic substance will probably not go amiss!

Sugar-cane

In 3,000 years sugar-cane (*see* fig 6.1) has, according to Stephen Harris, been transformed from a Papua New Guinean (PNG) 'kitchen garden' plant into a global 'agro-industrial' one! Before the *seventeenth* century, Europeans had very little, if any, experience of the sweetness of *sucrose* which in any case was hugely expensive; about half of today's *'refined-sugar'* is extracted from sugar-*cane*. Cane was described by John Gerard (1545–1612), the author of the popular *'Herball'* (1597) as a 'pleasant and profitable reed'. Cultivation requires a great deal of water and fertiliser (or fertile soil); therefore high rainfall, in addition to high ambient temperature is required, coupled with a high level of manual application.

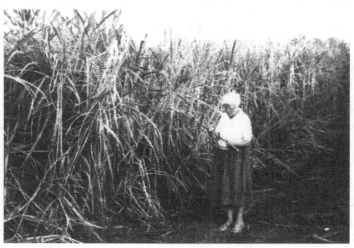

Fig 6.1: Sugar-cane grass (*see* Ref 1 [Duggan] 18).

The name of this genus of tropical and sub-tropical grass dates from Carolus Linnaeus (1707–98) who gave it the name *Saccharum*. As people migrated across Polynesia into southern and South East Asia, cane travelled with them, and by the *sixth* century it was grown in Persia (*now* Iran), and by the *eighth*, Egypt; by the *tenth* century it became an important Mediterranean crop. Arab expansion took cane throughout the Mediterranean area to the Iberian peninsula and by the *fifteenth* century both Spanish and Portuguese adventurers had introduced it to their Atlantic possessions. It was from there that it was transferred to the 'new world'.

The process of extraction and concentration of the sucrose content involves squeezing juice from the cane; after boiling, and as the concentrated juice cools, the sucrose crystallises while the molasses drains away. The sum total is that the equivalent of a field the size of a football pitch produces about 50 tonnes of cane with a resultant 6.5 tonnes of '*refined-sugar*'.

It was probably Christopher Columbus (1451–1506) who introduced sugar-cane from the Canary Islands to the 'new world' on his second voyage in 1492. He apparently supervised planting in Hispaniola (*now* the Dominican Republic) and Haiti (formerly the western part of Hispaniola). Iberian and British landowners then brought in Africans as slaves to work in the fields and thus the 'slave trade' (*see* below) was launched. The Englishman, a surgeon Benjamin Moseley (1742–1819) summarised the prevailing position in the *eighteenth* century:

> If Jamaica, and the other *English sugar islands*, were to share the fate of *St Domingue* [Haiti], by the horrors of war, a distress would arise, not only in England, but in Europe, not confined to the present generation, but that would descend to the child unborn. Of such important has the agriculture of half a million of Africans, become to Europeans.

It was during that century that the morality behind the trade became questioned, and it was early in the next that abolition was in people's minds. However, by this time Europeans had become addicted to '*refined-sugar*' (and were prepared to pay anything for it), despite the fact that dental problems and the 'pissing evil' (diabetes) were already associated with it. When its side-effects (*see* Chapters 10 and 11) *were* recognised, artificial sweeteners (*see* Chapter 14) – one being produced from the south American daisy *Stevia rebaudiana* (Aspartamine) – came into prominence! In *nineteenth* century Britain, as well as heralding origin(s) of the *Industrial Revolution*, numerous cities and buildings, etc, sugar-laden beverages – coffee, tea, and chocolate shops also escalated.

Sugar-beet

Stephen Harris claims that 'it was *sugar*-beet that promoted other forms of beet [in a wider sense] from a cottage garden vegetable to an industrial crop'.[1] In the *sixteenth* century, French cooks made sweet syrups from beetroot, and much later the German physicist Andreas Marggraf (1709–82) demonstrated that beetroot sugar was identical with cane-sugar – both consisting in fact largely of *sucrose*. However, by 1784, Franz Achard (1753–1821) began selective breeding of sugar-beet from white *Silesian marigolds*; he was backed by the Prussian government in the opening of a commercial factory for sugar beet extraction.

During the Napoleonic Wars (1805–15) access to the Caribbean, and hence acquisition of cane sugar ceased. It was Napoleon Bonaparte (1769–1821) himself who first attempted substitution of sugar-*beet* for sugar-*cane*. He had instructed a French chemist Antoine-Augustin Parmentier (1737–1813) to investigate the possibility of commercial extraction of sugar from sources other than sugar-cane; Parmentier concluded that beets were the best source. This was taken up by French industrialists, Jean-Baptiste Quéruel and Benjamin Defesseri. Between 1837 and 2010, France was the world's largest *sugar-beet* producer, and it also became part of Britain's agricultural landscape after the Great War (1914–18).

By 'selective breeding', sucrose content of sugar-beet rose from 5-6% (dry weight) to approximately 20%. Beet has the great advantage over cane that it flourishes in a low *temperate* climate, and can also be stored before sugar processing. Since the 1960s, annual worldwide sugar-beet production has reached 270 million tonnes, and now accounts for one third of the world's annual '*refined-sugar*' production. Furthermore, sugar-beet producers have begun exploring potential biofuels rather than fossil ones.

Historically, transition from honey to '*refined-sugar*' was a gradual process; while providing relatively low-priced calories for large sections of the world's human population, it became arguably responsible for more human disease than any other nutrient – one of which is of course *obesity* – the major *raison d'etre* of this book.

Origin of 'sugar' as a sweetener

The history of the place of origin of '*refined-sugar*' as *the* major sweetener has been admirably outlined in '*Sweetness and Power: The Place of sugar in Modern Society* (1985) by Sidney Mintz (1922–2015), a cultural anthropologist (*see* Chapter 5). *Sugar*-cane (from which most '*refined-sugar*' is presently derived) he concluded, probably originated in the southern Pacific, and arose during 'domestication' in *Papua New Guinea* and *Indonesia*. It was originally demonstrated that a 'crude kind of sugar could be obtained by extracting and drying the *sap* of sugar-cane'. From the Pacific region the tradition travelled to other tropical countries, including India, from whence it spread to China – the earliest reference to its cultivation dating to around 300 BC; however, with the growth of Buddhism its healing (not sweetness) ability (already appreciated in India), was widely accepted. By the *sixth* century AD, a *cane hybrid* reached Persia (now Iran), and by the *tenth* sugar-cane was an important *Middle Eastern* crop. As Arab expansion escalated more rapidly, cultivation spread around the Mediterranean, and by the *fifteenth* century, its growth was established in Madeira, as well as the *Canary* and *Cape Verde* islands, *São Tomé* and West Africa. By the mid-*eighteenth* century cane was cultivated in *Egypt*. Cane thrives in a hot climate, requires an abundance of water, and is intolerant of frost. Following harvesting, it is liquefied, boiled to honey-like molasses and refined syrup, and ultimately crystallised into household sugar. Although first stages of the process were almost certainly developed by various societies at different times, the more complex techniques leading to crystallised sugar probably originated from a single source in India and spread *via* trade routes – including the 'silk road' – ultimately reaching the *New World*.

At this point, 'refined-sugar' was beginning to overtake honey as a sweetener, and by the nineteenth century refining techniques had greatly improved. As early as 1633, a text by a Northampton physician – James

Hart (born c.1580) – predicted that 'sugar' would overtake honey because it was 'far more pleasing to the palate' and was also less allergenic! As late as the *eighteenth* century, sugar remained however, a very expensive luxury commodity throughout the world.

It took the Atlantic slave trade (see below) and resultant development of plantations in the Caribbean and South America to set a platform for today's sugar-industry.

John Yudkin (see Prologue) has emphasised the dissociation of palatability (ie, sweetness) from nutritional value (ie, vitamin content, etc); whereas in former times, essential nutrients such as vitamin C (ascorbic acid) had an origin in fruit and honey, the overriding contemporary requirement being sweetness, with little or no interest in essential nutrients.[2] The main focus of Yudkin's 1950s and 60s interest, as pointed out elsewhere in this book, was on its rôle in causing arterial disease (common in westernised society, and rapidly increasing in the 'third world') which has since become centred on dietary fibre and fat, unjustifiably shifting attention from the evils of 'refined-sugar'. The principal source of carbohydrate historically was of course starch, but this has been largely replaced by *'refined-sugar'*, starch barely figuring in a present day-to-day dietary.

There was, and remains, major finance in *'refined-sugar'* which is the main reason why it would certainly take legislation to reduce production – especially in infant foods, which must inevitably be sweet! Many consider, erroneously, that palatable foods are also nutritionally beneficial (and vice versa) – but that is of course far from the truth.

The transition from honey to 'refined-sugar'
Elizabeth Abbott in her excellent book: *Sugar: a bittersweet history* has provided a succinct historical account of the replacement of honey by *'refined-sugar'* as a *sweetener*. Alternative uses include:

- medicine for colds, sore throats, and menstrual discomfort,
- as a *spice* and *condiment,*
- as a *decorative* material, and
- as a preservative.

Unrefined cane has apparently also been used at various times as a building material, and its leaves have provided roofing material and also cattle fodder; cane *stalks* have been used historically as spears and occasionally splints; cane *sap* has even been used as a water source when drinking water is *not* readily available in the Third World, and rarely to remove evil spirits! Overall, uses have followed Arabic and Islamic culture geographically, and orientated around those irrigation techniques required for cane-growing.

REFINING

Little is known about ancient Arabic refining-techniques apart from the fact that they were obviously relatively unsophisticated, and probably arose at several sites independently. During the *eleventh* to *thirteenth* centuries, Christians participating in the *crusades* 'learned the art' of sugar-refining from Muslims, and they returned to Britain with a '*taste for sugar*'! In fact, the crusades laid foundations for sugar production and its use in Europe. When the 'Black Death' struck Europe in 1348–9, populations were decimated, and landowners thereafter employed Middle Eastern slaves to cultivate *sugar-cane* crops. Later, in the *fifteenth* century, Portuguese explorers introduced *sugar-cane* into West Africa and at that point the Atlantic slave trade (*see* below) had its origin.

Until about that time, sugar-refining had been carried out with a pair of grindstones – either human or animal powered. This was followed by boiling cane juice, while impurities were skimmed off before it was again boiled, poured into earthenware vessels and crystallised; the resultant molasses being again boiled to produce even more '*refined-sugar*'. The procedure was originally extremely expensive, and most produce was used to sweeten medicines. From the *fifteenth* century onwards, the process was carried out in refineries, frequently at a considerable distance from the site at which the cane was grown, *ie,* far away from the Middle East and Mediterranean.

Large scale '*refined-sugar*' *consumption* had its origin in royal and noble courts, and by the *sixteenth* century a connection between '*refined-sugar*' and '*power*' emerged. However, from then its price began to decline as increasing numbers of labourers became involved. When the 'new world' was 'discovered', sugar-cane planting began in earnest;

in Hispaniola (*now* Haiti) and the Dominican Republic colonists from Europe (principally Spain and Portugal), planted cane derived from the Canary Islands, and within a decade, scores of mills were processing cane, most for export to Spain, and sugar production in the 'new world' had really taken root. The *Sugar Islands* were then operative, and the triangular trade was destined to begin!

The Atlantic slave trade
Britain was a pioneer (and leader) in the early days of the West African trade; Sir John Hawkins (1532–95) became the first known British trader between 1562 and 67, and he made four voyages from Sierra Leone to Hispaniola; he sold his slaves to Spanish settlers. it is perhaps not widely appreciated that *'refined-sugar'* (from the *British Sugar Islands*), and more importantly its *production*, was the major *raison d'être* for the genesis of the Atlantic trade, its principal objective being to import cheap labour from Africa into the Caribbean and South America in order to grow and process cane for transport to Europe. Other crops were: cotton, tobacco, coffee, cocoa and rice. Slavery was of course *not* new to Africa[3], for within the continent it had certainly existed for several centuries; trade between Africa and Asia had also existed for several millennia, accurate documentation existing from the *seventh* century. Trade between *West* Africa and the 'new world' began in the *sixteenth* century and continued well into the *nineteenth* (*ie,* a period of more than three hundred years). The 'slave coast' extended from present-day Ivory Coast to Nigeria, whilst the 'triangular trade' (most centred on Liverpool) rapidly developed:

- The *first* 'leg' was organised to transport guns, gunpowder, and cowrie shells (collected from the Indian Ocean), glass beads, iron rods or bars and manillas (a primitive form of currency) to West Africa; ships also carried a few passengers – most of them replacement staff for West African forts – many built and manned by Portuguese, and some by the British who established and managed them *via* the *Royal Africa Company*, or local administrative centres. Although also used to house slaves, they were originally built to trade with interior states,

- The *second* 'leg' (the 'middle passage') carried African *slaves* – under incredibly cramped and immoral conditions, to either the Caribbean or South America. It is estimated that during some 35,000 voyages, 10.7 million West Africans were transported. Prior to 1750, the emphasis was on the Caribbean, and after that, Brazil became the major 'target', Spain and Portugal being the major transporters. Ships also carried gold and ivory (which often ultimately reached Britain), and occasionally African cloth and metalwork. Disease and mortality, as is widely known, were rife on these voyages, and
- The *third* (and final 'leg') of the triangular trade, brought the ships back to Britain or another European country; they transported produce from the Caribbean, South America, and (to a lesser extent) north American countries.

'*Refined-sugar*', coffee, cocoa, cotton and tobacco were all carried to Britain where they helped boost the national economy.[4]

A recently published novel: *Willoughbyland* (2015) gives a vivid description of the industry. In the *seventeenth* century, Sir Walter Raleigh (1552–1618) was heavily involved in expeditions to the Spanish Main – especially the Suriname River area (present-day Guyana), with a view to expanding Britain's overseas empire. These ambitions however came to nought, but the following governor of nearby Barbadoes (now Barbados) and later Governor of the Caribbees was Lord Francis Willoughby (1613–66) who had other ideas. Although various commodities – including gold – remained tempting, especially in the mythical land of El Dorado, he decided to explore '*refined-sugar*' production (tobacco and cotton were alternatives which were later abandoned), which he considered would boost the wealth of the rapidly expanding British Empire. Sugar at Willoughbyland was apparently superior to that in Barbadoes! The subject of *sugar,* and particularly expansion of African slavery (henceforth more profitable than gold) was brought to the fore in a *seventeenth* century novel (*Oroonoko*) (later to become one of the most popular dramas of the British theatrical repertory of the 1700s) written by Aphra Behn (1640–89) and subsequently a favourite book of the abolitionists.[5] African labour was already well established in Barbadoes and other West Indian territories, and the appalling conditions here were no better![6] The immensely profitable British sugar colony of Suriname – belonging to Willoughby – was eventually obliterated following both an epidemic and various battles involving French and subsequently Dutch troops. Meanwhile, Willoughby's descendant, William (by then Governor of the Caribbees) continued with the sugar industry, but in Barbadoes rather than Willoughbyland.[7]

Treatment of slaves *in the* 'new *world'*

Before the African trade became operative, Spaniards had apparently attempted to enslave local Amerindians, but for various reasons this policy failed. Newly arrived slaves from West Africa were either taken straight to a plantation, or to a slave-market provided they had not already been sold (as most had). Existent slaves, of whom their owners were anxious to dispose, were also subjected to this humiliating experience. However, sale in a slave-market was expensive, and many were therefore purchased *via* advertisements in local newspapers. Slaves were employed in various capacities, depending largely upon age. Not all were channelled to a plantation, some being employed as domestic servants, or directed to other occupations; in Brazil, for example, gold mining became the major economy, and other enslaved workers participated in building an urban society, while many became skilled craftsmen, *eg,* builders, blacksmiths or carpenters.

Development of the *new world* was thus based on a plantation economy in which everyone knew his/her place in society. Estates were managed by a plantation owner, whose wife in most cases looked after both house and *domestic* 'enslaved' labour. On larger plantations, an *overseer* undertook management of the plantation, and in some cases several trusted 'enslaved' workers became slave-drivers. At the base of the pyramid was the 'enslaved' labourer who simply had absolutely no individual rights. The plantation owner often had sexual relations with his female slaves, and hence mixed-race children resulted; they were in consequence often either *not* accepted or well treated by the owner's wife! Major plantations in the Caribbean, USA and South America (especially Brazil) grew not only sugar, but also cotton, coffee, tobacco, rice and cocoa. Livestock was also kept to provide sustenance for 'enslaved' workers.

Obviously a great deal of antagonism often emerged between the 'enslaved' and owner – amounting in some cases to uprisings and rebellion. In Hispaniola, for example, a major revolt began in 1791 and was of such magnitude that British, French and Spanish authorities each sent forces in an attempt to terminate this rebellion; a local statesman who sided with the French, was ultimately arrested and deported to France where he later died. There were numerous other examples of unrest in the Caribbean and South America (Brazil being an important focus) and the USA. Many slaves escaped – some in groups – while others assisted by local people who opposed slavery, thus risked arrest or occasionally more serious consequences. Some slaves ultimately reached Europe – transported by either a plantation-owner or a ship's captain – to whom possession of a *black* servant was often a valuable prestige symbol. If sent to the Caribbean however, they were usually returned to slavery but some, *eg,* Ignatius Sancho (1729–80) and Olaudah Equiano (1745–97)[8], eventually gained freedom in England.

EMANCIPATION
Although the founder of the Quaker movement – George Fox (1624–91) – was strongly opposed to slavery, the *Society for the Abolition of the Slave Trade* in Britain was not formed until 1787 (also by the Quakers) with the collaboration of two Anglican churchmen (Granville Sharp and Thomas Clarkson), with William Wilberforce ([1759–1833]) as their parliamentary spokesman. This Society obviously received strong support from Africans in Britain (*see* above), some of whom had 'escaped' from southern America; they believed that Atlantic slavery should be abolished and replaced by *employed* labour. British abolitionists subsequently developed Freetown (Sierra Leone) for both repatriated and 'rescued' Africans who wished to re-establish their lives in Africa.

In Britain, a boycott of *'refined-sugar'* began in 1792, when about 300,000 people abandoned it as a household commodity! The abolitionists, led by Wilberforce in parliamentary debates, however, demanded legislation *against* the trade which they claimed was 'contrary to the principles of Christianity, justice, humanity and sound policy'; this resulted in passing of the *'Slave Trade* Bill' of 1807 by both houses of Parliament, abolishing *British* involvement in the trade, but *not* slavery itself. Between 1808 and 1888, Royal Navy (RN) patrols (in the West Africa squadron) freed approximately 150,000 'enslaved' Africans from 1,600 slave-ships, most being returned to West Africa – usually Sierra Leone. The British had therefore taken a major part in both establishment and later abolition of the Atlantic trade.

But *legislation* had failed to go far enough, for slavery remained intact in British territories, albeit to a lesser extent. In 1823 the *Anti-Slavery Society* was founded – with Clarkson and Wilberforce at its helm. Because women were excluded from this society, *The Ladies Society for the Relief of Negro Slaves* was formed in 1825. Several prominent individuals in Britain – including Admiral Lord Nelson (1758–1805) were, however, themselves slave-owners who staunchly *opposed* abolition. However, in 1833 the British government passed a Bill – which became law on 1 August the following year – outlawing slavery in *all* British territories, slave-owners receiving £12 per slave (£20 million in all). The 'enslaved' workers however, did *not* receive compensation or an immediate advantage other than being free to seek employment elsewhere.

Despite these developments in Britain, slavery continued in many other parts of the world, and in 1839 the *British and Foreign Anti-Slavery Society* was formed as a result. In the USA, Atlantic anti-slavery *legislation* was also supported by Quakers, and came to fruition in 1808. America established its own colony – Liberia – in 1821–2, and numerous freed slaves were repatriated to that country. Some former African slaves, however remained in the USA, and in 1851 Harriet Beecher Stowe (1811–96)'s famous novel *Uncle Tom's Cabin*[9] was first published. Cuba abolished slavery in 1886, and Brazil (the last in the western hemisphere to do so) two years later.

LEGACIES OF THE TRADE

The Atlantic trade left several legacies – some good and others despicable, many being still visible in America, Europe and even Africa. On the *positive* side may be placed anti-racism, architectural developments, business and finance, and cultural diversity. On a *negative* side however, West Africa was depleted of much of her population – especially young adults; this therefore retarded African progress and development, and allowed western powers to fight, unopposed, over natural resources (including oil), exploitation of palm oil, cocoa, gold and timber. An important outcome was the 'scramble for Africa' in the aftermath of World War I (1914–18), accompanied by carving up of a large part of the continent by European powers, much with imposition of *artificial* national boundaries. This era, as Abbott has admirably narrated in her book, must be held to some extent responsible for many of today's West African problems.[10]

Problems resulting from the slave trade had *not* of course in the *twentieth* century been entirely solved. Other legacies arose much later, and threats of *legislation* persist, *eg,* the then British Prime Minister – David Cameron – visited Jamaica in 2015 and was asked by the 'reigning' Jamaican Prime Minister – Ms Portia Simpson-Miller – to apologise for Britain's role in the trade. In response Cameron announced a £25 million donation in order to establish a prison on that Caribbean island, to which Jamaican prisoners numbering >600 in British jails, would be repatriated from Britain.[11]

Another example of a long-term enigma relates to the reputation of Edward Colston (1636–1721), a benefactor of numerous charities, etc in Bristol, England, and commemorated by a window in the cathedral. Most of his wealth was apparently generated from the slave trade however, and questions currently being asked in 2017 are: (i) should he be remembered as a slave trader *or* beneficiary, and (ii) should the window in Bristol Cathedral be removed?[12] A similar campaign is in progress at Liverpool, but here William Gladstone (1809–98) is the victim.[13]

In **conclusion**, production of '*refined-sugar*' has in recent years escalated and this has now become one of the world's major manufacturing industries. This produce now provides cheap calories for much of the growing world population, and it is now difficult to foresee a day when the world's calorie-source outstrips the rapidly increasing population as forecast by Thomas Robert Malthus [(1766–1834)], the *seventeenth* century British economist. Surely mere awareness of the awful reputation of this history should inculcate a sense of profound repugnance of this obnoxious trade and its resultant product – '*refined-sugar*'.

References and notes

1   S Harris. *What have plants ever done for us?* Oxford: Bodleian Library 2015: 20–3, 178–82; M Duggan. *Sugar for the House: a history of early sugar refining in north west England.* London: Fonthill Media Ltd 2013: 175.

2   Anonymous. Sidney Mintz. Food anthropologist who traced the origins of Britain's love of sugar. *Times, Lond* 2016; January 5: 54; J Yudkin. *Pure, white and deadly: how sugar is killing us and what we can do to stop it.* London: Penguin Books 1986: 200;

3   M Park. *Travels in the interior of Africa.* London: Wordsworth 2002: 406; M Duttill. *Mungo Park* Edinburgh, Scotland: NHS Publishing 1999: 144.

4   E Abbott. *Sugar: a bittersweet history.* London: Duckworth Overlook 2010: 453. (*See also*: H Thomas. *The Slave trade: the history of the Atlantic slave trade 1440–1870.* London: Picador 1997: 925; N Sadler. *The Slave Trade.* London; Shire Publications 2009: 64; A Stuart. *Sugar in the Blood: a family's story of slavery and empire.* London: Portobello Books 2012: 424; D Olusoga. *Black and British: a forgotten history.* London: MacMillan 2016: 602; J Walvin. *Sugar: the world corrupted, from slavery to obesity.* London: Robinson 2017: 325; J T Cathey, J S Marr. Yellow fever, Asia and the East African slave trade. *Trans R Soc trop Med Hyg* 2014; 108: 252–7.

5   A Behn. *Oroonoko, or the Royal Slave: a true history.* London; W Canning 1688.

6   Op cit. *See* note 4 above.

7   M Parker. *Willoughbyland: England's lost colony.* London: Hutchinson 2015: 294.

8   R King. *Ignatius Sancho: an African man of letters.* London: National Portrait Gallery 1997: 17; O Equiano: *The Interesting Narrative and other writings.* London; Penguin Books 1995: 355; I Sancho. *Letters of the late Ignatius Sancho, an African.* London: Penguin Books 1998.

9   H B Stowe. *Uncle Tom's Cabin: or Life among the Lowly.* London; Penguin Books 1986: 629; Anonymous. (On this day). London celebrates the end of slavery. *Times, Lond* 2000; August 2: 2; D Stevenson. A history of slavery: facts and fallacies. *Ibid* 2015: October 5: 28.

10 Op cit. *See* note 4 above.

11 F Gibb. Two centuries on, Caribbean leaders prepare to sue Britain over slave trade. *Times, Lond* 2014; March 10: 3; D Wilson. Caribbean nations and the effects of slavery. *Ibid* 2014: March 12: 29; S Sherlock. Slavery's legacy. *Ibid* 2013; November 28: 29; F Karim. £25m deal to return Jamaican prisoners. *Ibid* 2015: September 30: 2; T Hunt. We shouldn't pay blood money for slavery: instead of historical apologies we ought to use our aid budget to boost cultural and educational links to the Caribbean. *Ibid* 2015; October 3: 28.

12 Anonymous. Slave to the Past: changing the name of Colston's Hall in Bristol will not change history. *Ibid* 2017; April 27:23; L Bannerman, R Morrison. Concert Hall is renamed to end slave trade link. *Ibid* 2017; April 27: 17; R Bennett. Girls' school keeps name of founding slave trader. *Ibid* 2017; November 3: 15.

13 R Bennett. Students want Gladstone name dropped from halls. *Ibid* 2017; November 16: 6.

14 J Root. Stain of slavery. *Ibid* 2017; February 23: 28; S Bush. Anti-slavery patrols. *Ibid* 2017; February 24: 28; P James. Population Malthus: his life and times. London: Routledge and Kegan Paul 1979: 524.

PART II:

Metabolism and *clinical* consequences of excessive dietary sugar and obesity

CHAPTER 7:

How much 'refined-sugar' (sucrose) are we ingesting in 2017?

Average northern European diets, in this author's opinion, contain far too many calories derived from 'refined-sugar', with corresponding exclusion of healthy food – *ie,* fruit and vegetables. Therefore an ideal 'Mediterranean diet' is becoming extremely unusual in Britain (*see also* Chapter 12). The principal *raison d'être* of this chapter therefore is to separate a 'healthy' diet, whatever the cause of obesity transpires to be, from an unhealthy one, acknowledging that being overweight must ultimately be caused by an imbalance between input and output of calories, however derived.

Healthy diets in history
A fascinating investigation, perhaps not directly relevant to present-day humans, has focused on dietary methods to avoid/counteract obesity. The diet of a cave-woman (Palaeolithic[¶]) was the focus of an *MRC Epidemiological Unit* study at Cambridge, the results of which were published in the *European Journal of Clinical Nutrition*. Diet consisted of: berries, vegetables, and lean meat – which over three weeks had already been shown to reduce incidence of both myocardial infarction and stroke in men. Seventy 'heavily overweight women' were placed on either this diet or alternatively a modern European one; after six months on the 'cave-woman diet' the women lost on average 6.2 kg, while waist circumferences had reduced by a mean of 11 cm, and comparable figures for those on the 'modern European' diet were 2.6 kg and 5.8 cm, respectively.[1]

The *Health Survey for England* analysed dietary data from 65,000 people: 4,300 had died during an eight-year follow-up period, risk of death depending largely on frequency of consumption of fruit and

---

[¶] The *Palaeolithic period* extended from 2.6 million until about 10,000 years ago in Europe and the Middle East. The term was coined by the archaeologist John (later 1st Baron Avebury) Lubbock (1834–1913) in 1865. (J Owen. *Darwin's Apprentice: An archaeological biography of John Lubbock.* London : Pen and Sword Archaeology 2013 : 177.)

vegetables; cardiac disease and 'cancer' were also significantly reduced (*see also* Chapter 11). Seven portions of fruit and vegetables daily (*see* Chapter 12) reduced risk of early death by 42%, suggesting that *five* portions daily – recommended by the *National Health Service* (NHS) – might be insufficient! This 'five-a-day' diet presupposes, of course, that a 'healthy' diet does *not* contain significant quantities of added '*refined-sugar*'. A *Sunday Times* article indicated that most dietary items are in fact 'packed with sugar'.[2] *One* to *three*, and *three* to *five* portions daily were accompanied by reduced mortality rates of 15% and 36%, respectively. Vegetables were more effective than fruit, possibly because small amounts of fructose in the latter render it relatively counter-productive, although potentially desirable; effect of the *fructose* component seems *not* to have been considered. Perhaps therefore, the ideal frequency of vegetables/ fruit should be as much as *ten* portions daily![3]

Present-day foodstuffs

In contrast to *historical* times (*see* above), most present-day 'industrial-ised' foods contain a significant quantity of '*refined-sugar*', even though its presence is often far from obvious. According to the London *Times* newspaper, weight of added '*refined-sugar*' (sucrose) (g/100g) in UK breakfast cereals (*see also* Chapter 3) is as shown in Table 7.1. An article in London's *Sunday Times* concluded that even so-called '*healthy* break-fast biscuits and cereal bars' contain 'up to 42% sugar', the worst being *Kellogg's Coco Pops* snack bar. In an attempt to make products appear more healthy, the food industry has decided to advertise their cereals as 'bursting' with fruit, or in other cases 'seriously fruity' or even 'over-flowing with tangy blackcurrants, blueberries, cranberries and crunchy almonds'. However, researchers for that newspaper concluded that these cereals, as well as containing 'high levels of sugar' were accompanied by 'as little as 3% fruit'! There is no doubt that most '*refined-sugar*' concen-trations – especially in children's cereals – are high.[4] Other relevant arti-cles have given 'sugar' content of numerous day-to-day dietary items, in many of which the '*refined-sugar*' content (and probably that of artificial sweeteners also) is far too high.[5]

Table 7.1: Weight of *'refined-sugar'* (g/100g) in UK breakfast cereals

Shredded Wheat	0.7
Scott's Porage Oats	1.0
Weetabix	4.4
Kellogg's Cornflakes	8.0
Rice Krispies	10.0
Essential Waitrose Wholegrain Bran Flakes	17.0
Jordan's Super Berry Granola	20.1
Nestlé Cheerios	21.4
Special K Red Berries	22.0
Sugar Puffs	35.0
Kellogg's Coco Pops	35.0

'Fizzy' (sugary) drinks

The case against *sugar-containing* drinks has also been admirably summarised by the *Times* health correspondent:

> Even one *Coke* is too many. A can of *Coca-Cola* contains 33g of sugar – about *six* teaspoonsful – and in July 2015 the government's scientific advisory committee on nutrition halved its recommendation on sugar intake, saying we should get no more than 5 per cent of *daily* calories from sugar, *i.e.*, the equivalent of about 30g. The average British adult consumes about twice that amount, so it is hardly surprising [that] most of us are overweight.
>
> Is sugar uniquely evil? The US endocrinologist Robert Lustig says *the body processes sugar differently and each calorie of sugar is more likely to make us fat than a calorie of other foods* [my italics]. The scientific consensus tends to disagree. The same review found no specific link between *'refined-sugar'* and many of the most common diseases, though it said that people who drank more *sugary drinks* were more likely to get *type-2-diabetes*.
>
> Instead, the crucial finding was that if you eat more sugar, you eat more, full stop. In other words, people who eat more

sugar do not cut out other foods to compensate. It is this extra weight that leads to high blood pressure, cancer, heart disease and a range of other killers [*see* Chapter 11].

In this respect sugar is unusual. Although scientists are not sure why, there is one obvious explanation: if you eat a hamburger, you feel full, [but if] you drink a *Coke*, you don't. You're therefore more likely to have another one – and a hamburger as well.[6]

Drinks targeted at children, which contain far too much '*refined-sugar*' have rightly come in for a great deal of media attention; *Coca-Cola* in particular received criticism.[7] '*Refined-sugar*' (and other components) from several sauces were tabulated by *Times 2* in early 2016 (*see* Table 7.2).[8]

Table 7.2: Sauces recommended to be eaten only *once* weekly[**]

Sauce (title/brand)	Weight (g per 100g) or calories per 100g			
	Refined sugar	Fat	Salt	Calories
Uncle Ben's sweet and sour	16.2	0.2	0.43	85
Dolmio Bolognese	5.8	0.6	0.80	44
Tesco Finest black bean	0.7	2.1	0.70	114
Jamie Oliver tomato and Italian red wine	5.3	2.7	0.83	67
Seeds of Change organic Mediterranean vegetables Pasta	6.3	2.9	0.64	60
Dolmio Bolognese pasta	4.2	0.10	0.80	33
Newman's Own Bastilico pasta	10.6	1.5	0.80	70
Dolmio Cheesy – for lasagne	2.3	8.1	0.80	102
Spice Tailor tikka masala	6.4	14.2	1.30	180
Tesco Bolognese pasta	7.3	0.3	0.70	42
Loyd Grossman Bolognese	5.2	2.5	0.82	55
Homepride bake creamy tomato and herb	5.8	7.4	0.84	106
Waitrose half fat biryani	4.9	2.9	0.48	58
Dolmio classic basil	3.3	52	1.40	511.1
Newman's Own Bolognese	9.7	2.1	0.80	71
Dolmio tomato red lasagne	6.4	0.2	0.82	47
Waitrose rogan josh	4.9	21.2	2.48	249
Seeds of change organic tomato and basil	6.9	2.9	0.65	63
Loyd Grossman tikka masala	9.0	10.6	0.85	147
Louis Martin chair de tomate with basil	4.2	1.6	1.00	47

[**] *See: Times 2, Lond* 2016: April 18: 7 and ref 8.

Healthy eating

A later article in London's *Sunday Times* newspaper indicated, that 'Food companies are [both] surprisingly and dishonestly utilising a government-backed campaign [in order] to persuade [readers] to eat more healthily [and to] sell less products laden with sugar'. This *'five-a-day'* promotion (*see* above) is based on advice provided by the *World Health Organisation* (WHO) recommendation of a daily minimum of 400g of fruit and vegetables, or alternatively five portions of 80g of each, in order to lower incidence of diseases including: *obesity*, arterial disease, and type-2-diabetes. Some of these products consist of three-quarters *'refined-sugar'*. Examples of dietary components with a range varying from 49–83% 'sugar' were provided – many targeting children!

In mid-2014 the same newspaper also published details of the colossal amounts of *'refined-sugar'* in certain 'fast foods'. A review of 'ready meals' from *six* of Britain's supermarkets revealed that some contained *more* sugar than the daily recommended limit of 50g (or 25g according to 'draft guidelines' from the *WHO*) laid down by *Public Health England* . The worst quoted was *Sainsbury*'s 'Sweet and Sour Chicken with Rice' a pack of which apparently contains 50.7g (equivalent to *ten* teaspoonfuls) of *'refined-sugar'*.[9] An investigation involving 17 'ready meals' obtained from major supermarkets also found the highest 'sugar' content to be in 'sweet and sour' dishes; many containing more sugar than the recommended limit of 50g as in an adult's daily intake, and about twice that of a standard *Dairy Milk chocolate bar*.[10] In another study it was shown that *low*-fat food products are more likely to contain added 'sugar' than those with a *full*-fat content; however, they possess 'at least as many calories'; because manufacturers apparently tend to use extra 'sugar' to counteract loss of taste resulting from reduced fat content. A further study, presented to the *European Congress on Obesity,* referred to the very high concentration of 'sugar' in *white* bread – again apparently leading to an increased risk of obesity.[11]

Table 7.3: Best 'healthy' vegetables (and recommended daily intake) – based on a 'seven-a-day' intake.

	Quantity per single portion††
Kale	Four teaspoons (cooked)
Watermelon	Large slice
Beetroot	80g
Watercress	85g
Carrots	Two
Kiwi fruit	One
Onions	One
Yellow peppers	Half
Jerusalem artichokes	80g
Papaya	One
Tomatoes	One
Broccoli	Three florets
Blueberries	Small handful
Cucumber	One quarter

Table 7.4 – Twelve fruits and vegetables for consumption at least once weekly, and their health benefits‡‡

Food	Active constituent	Health benefit
Raspberries	Antioxidants/ellagicacid/ manganese	Anti-carcinogenic/maintains bone density
Rocket	Nitrates/folate	Hypotensive/haematinic
Salmon	Omega-3 fatty acids	Boosts memory/vision Hypotensive/cardiogenic
Turmeric	Curcumin	Anti-inflammatory/arthritis
Brazil nuts	Selenium	Prostate cancer
Shitake mushrooms	Vitamin D	Enhances bone density/boosts immune function
Tomatoes	Lycopene	Antioxidant/prostate disease
Walnuts	Antioxidant/Omega 3 fatty acids	Prevention of myocardial infarction and diabetes
Miso (soya beans)	Lactic acid	Maintenance of colonic bacteria
Garlic	Allicin	Cholesterol lowering/ anti-inflammation/anti-atherogenic
Pineapple		Mucus reduction/muscle & joint repair/anticoagulant
Avocado	Potassium/Vitamins K and E/ mono-unsaturated fats	Hypotension/anticoagulant

---

†† *See Times 2, Lond* 2014 ; April 2: 3, and ref 3 (Bee)
‡‡ *See Times 2, Lond* 2016 ; July 2 : 8, and ref 12 (Marber)

ACCEPTABLE FOODSTUFFS

It is therefore clear that many present-day foodstuffs contain a huge excess of *'refined-sugar'* coupled with far too little fruit and vegetables. In two recent articles, the 14 'best' vegetables (several portions daily) to counteract obesity have been analysed and shown to be *excellent* health foods. Most vegetables also contain significant concentrations of vitamins – the quantities of which obviously differ in various species. In addition, these articles contain advice on benefits of each item, as well as 'quick dishes' and various 'top tips'. The other article outlines 12 vegetable/fruit foods which do *not* contain *'refined-sugar'* and are strongly recommended for healthy eating (*see* tables 7.3 and 7.4)[12]

Correspondence in the *Times* newspaper in 2014 reminded its senior readership that in school photographs from the 1950s there are *no* children suffering from obesity. Now, (in 2014–2017) there is also absolutely *no* evidence of children walking or cycling to or from school, and also that tracks on common land have returned to grass through lack of use![13]

Other unhealthy foodstuffs

This chapter has alluded to dietary items containing an excess of *'refined-sugar'* and also *healthy* fruit and vegetables. It was recently revealed that Pope Francis (1936–present) – the 266th pontiff – had in 2015 been advised to eat less pasta (opinion is divided on whether that is obesogenic or not), and to take more exercise; he is also apparently fond of desserts (most containing a high concentration of *'refined-sugar'*). It seems difficult, however, to appreciate how pasta fits into a 'Mediterranean diet'![14]

Laboratory tests have recently been undertaken on *Diet Coke* and *Diet Pepsi*, in both of which very high concentrations of caffeine were discovered, compared with those in *regular Coke* and Pepsi. While there is now a requirement for 'fizzy drink' manufacturers to disclose the concentration of *'refined-sugar'* (sucrose), there is apparently no such regulation for caffeine.[15]

DISPOSAL OF EXCESS CALORIES

An interesting and useful table (*see* table 7.5) was published in January 2016, which indicates the amount of exercise required to 'burn off' the *excess* of dietary calories consumed in food.

Table 7.5: Duration of exercise required to metabolise ('burn off') an excess of calories contained in some foodstuffs[§§]

Nature of meal	Calorie content	Duration of exercise (min)	
		Walking	Running
Fruit and nut selection (200g)	972	179	67
Pret a Manger Swedish meatball wrap	636	115	43
Krispy Kreme caramel doughnut	397	73	27
Snickers	296	55	25
McCoy's cheddar and onion crisps (50g)	262	32	12
Cadbury Crème Egg	177	32	12
McVitie's digestive biscuit	71	13	5
Pizza Express American hot pizza	807	150	55
M&S ham, cheese and pickle sandwich	504	92	35
Chicken Caesar salad	361	66	25
Sainsbury's Belgian chocolate cake	282	54	20
Starbuck's grande flat white	220	40	15
Tropicana Smooth juice (300 ml)	144	27	10
Nairn's fine milled oatcake	36	6	2
Triple-layer carrot cake (slice)	655	120	45
Sharwood's prawn crackers (60g)	316	60	22
Tesco sushi, large fish selection	376	68	25
Tesco Snack classic pork pie (65g)	240	49	18
Coca-Cola (500 ml)	210	38	14
Müllerlight Greek lemon yoghurt	107	19	7
Banana	53	11	4

OTHER NUTRITIONAL MATTERS

Food labelling

The amount of *'refined-sugar'* added to a food item is often heavily disguised by the manufacturers, and consequently labels frequently contain highly confused information. A *single* portion of processed food can, for example, contain *more* than that recommended for an entire day. Percentage recommended on a label daily for an adult is based on the total sugar limit, rather than the strict limit on added sugar, a move which apparently renders product information completely meaningless and valueless.[16]

When the *Department of Health* launched their *'five-a-day'* scheme (*see* above), it recommended that food manufacturers should *not* use

[§§] Calculations based on 35-year-old man weighing 12.0 stone [76 kg]. *See: Times 2, Lond* 2016: January 18: 7.

their own logo 'on products aimed at children, or on (any food or drink) containing added sugar or salt'. Manufactures however, craftily avoided this recommendation by placing their *own 'five-a-day'* labels on products containing high concentrations of sugar and salt, and focused merely on a minority of acceptable nutrients.[17]

Discarded food

There has recently, quite rightly, been a great deal of attention to discarded and therefore *wasted* food in Britain (*see* Preface); only two per cent of 340,000 tonnes of surplus food produced by retailers, manufacturers and suppliers is currently redistributed. It is noteworthy that in a breakdown of waste, 21% represents fruit and vegetables, but 'fast foods' rank far lower! Again, this points to the fact that more nutritionally valuable items are discarded.[18]

Conclusion

Overall, what we eat is constantly moulding our bodies, including weight – and obesity. By eating nutritional foodstuffs rather than food loaded with *'refined-sugar'* and too few vitamins, the most disastrous disease in the world – *obesity* – could be totally avoided. This chapter has also given some guidance on what constitutes a *healthy* diet! But at last there is limited evidence that the major food companies have begun reducing *refined-sugar* in breakfast cereals.[19]

References and notes

1   Anonymous. Eat like a cavewoman to lose weight fast. *Times, Lond* 2014; April 2: 13. (*See also*: G Coren. Could a caveman diet cure the curse of the Corens? *Times 2, Lond* 2015; March 17: 4–5; O Moody. Think carefully before returning to Stone Age diet. *Times, Lond* 2015; August 12: 15; Anonymous. Paleo diet was a veggie feast with a side of meat. *New Scientist* 2016; December 10: 7.)

2   K Mansey. 'Five-a-day' foods packed with sugar. *Sunday Times, Lond* 2014; January 12: 5. (*See also*: K Lay. Fruit juices are too sugary to be included in five-a-day. *Times, Lond* 2014; November 11: 7.)

3   C Smyth. Five a day might not be enough to keep doctor away. *Ibid* 2014; April 1: 16; P Bee. The super fruit and veg guide. *Times 2, Lond* 2014; 2 April: 5; H Wallop. Do crisps count? How I survived a week on a 10-a-day diet: scientists say it's a regimen that could extend the lives of millions. *Ibid* 2017: April 13: 4–5.

4   H Rumbelow. How can you stop your kids from getting caned on sugar? *Times, Lond* 2014; January 9: 4–5; J Ungoed-Thomas, V Bennett. 'Healthy' cereals mix high sugar with little fruit. *Sunday Times, Lond* 2014; December 7: 17; P Ellis. Sugar-packed cereals making us fat. *Ibid* 2014; December 14: 34; K Lay. Breakfast cereal as sugary as seven chocolate biscuits. *Times, Lond* 2015; January 28: 24; B Earl, J Ungoed-Thomas. 'Healthy' cereal bars chewed out over sugar levels. *Sunday Times, Lond* 2015; March 15: 16.

5   Anonymous. Check your sugar intake: how much are you really eating? *Times, Lond* 2014; January 25: 12–13; Anonymous. The Good Sugar Guide. *Ibid* 2014; March 8: 20; H Summers. Ready meal has double the sugar of chocolate bar. *Sunday Times, Lond* 2014; May 18: 6; O Moody. Fruit snacks aimed at children contain more sugar than sweets. *Times, Lond* 2015; May 29: 17; P Bee. Hold the gourmet popcorn: is there such a thing as a healthy snack? *Times 2, Lond* 2015: August 10: 4–5. (*See also*: C Midgley. Two weeks on a low-fat diet ruined my liver. *Ibid;* June 29: 6–7; A Ellson. More pasta sauces need sugar and fat warnings, say experts. *Times, Lond* 2016; April 16: 9.)

6   Anonymous. Soft drinks less sugary abroad than in Britain. *Ibid* 2015; October 1: 19; D Lomas. Coca-cola and the debate about sugar. *Ibid* 2015; October 10: 24; S Griffiths. Jamie's restaurants cut fizzy drink

consumption with 10p sugar tax. *Sunday Times, Lond* 2015; October 18: 15; P Kidd. Once more unto the breach with Jamie in the battle of sugar hill. *Times, Lond* 2015; October 20: 17; Anonymous. Fizzy drink could deliver knockout blow to tumours. *Ibid* 2016: June 8: 18; O Moody. Why sugar-free drinks tempt you into eating bigger meals. *Ibid* 2016; December 14: 19; C Smyth. Diet drinks no healthier than sugary versions, scientists warn. *Ibid* 2017; January 4: 1,4. (*See also*: Chapter 14.)

7   K Lay. The sweet path to being obese. *Ibid* 2014; October 9: 8.

8   Anonymous. So should we eat these only once a week? *Times 2, Lond* 2016: April 18: 7.

9   K Mansey. 'Five-a-day' foods packed with sugar. *Sunday Times, Lond* 2014; January 12:5; Op cit. *See* note 5 (Summers) above.

10 *Ibid.*

11 O Moody. Beware the calories in low-fat foods. *Times, Lond* 2014; May 30: 16.

12 Op cit. *See* note 3 (Bee) above; Anonymous. Guess how many hours it takes to work off that treat! *Times 2, Lond* 2015; January 18: 7; I Marber. The 12 foods to eat every week. *Times 2, Lond* 2016; July 2: 8; P Bee. Fad or fab? What nutritionists say about the new super-foods: from a Siberian fungus to a Peruvian radish, sales of these fashionable dietary supplements have shot up. But are these so-called 'superfoods' worth buying? *Ibid* 2015; February 28: 6–7. (*See also*: P Bee. The end of fruit? How it became a guilt food: because of the nutritional war on sugar, fruit is being demonised. *Ibid* 2015; April 20: 6–7; A Maxted. Pick and mix – how to give your weekly shop a health kick. *Ibid* 2017; April 3: 4–5.)

13 J Anslow. Obesity? We have only ourselves to blame. *Times, Lond* 2014; January 15: 25.

14 P Willan. 'Unhealthy' Pope told to cut down on pasta. *Ibid* 2015; April 2: 47; O Moody. Pasta makes you slim, say (Italian) scientists. *Ibid* 2016; July 5: 15.

15 K Mansey. Tests reveal extra shot of caffeine in Diet Cola. *Sunday Times, Lond* 2014; August 3: 7.

16 J Ungoed-Thomas, J Boswell. Food labelling hides true scale of sugar hit. *Ibid* 2015: August 2: 6.

17 K Gibbons. Duchy dessert has twice the sugar of other brands. *Times, Lond* 2016; October 26: 7; (*See also*: C Smyth. Food giants reject lower sugar target. *Ibid* 2017; March 22: 1, 2; Anonymous. Sweet Nothings: if food manufacturers will not agree to cut sugar, the government must make them. *Ibid* 2017; March 22: 27.M Savage. Supermarkets told to give more food to those in need. *Ibid* 2014; June 2: 5; B Webster. Families bin good food on supermarket advice. *Ibid* 2017; February 27: 6; Anonymous. Waste Not: your nose knows best. *Ibid;* February 27: 29; B Webster. Scrap use-by dates on milk to end waste of 100 million pints. *Ibid* 2017; February 27: 1.

18 K Lay. Kellogg's to reduce sugar in top cereals. *Ibid* 2017; December 1: 17.

CHAPTER 8:

Fructose absorption and metabolism in *Homo sapiens*: in what form does *'refined-sugar'* (sucrose) enter the human portal circulation and liver?

This chapter focuses on the absorption products of *'refined-sugar'* (sucrose) in *Homo sapiens*. This author strongly believes that owing to its entrance into the portal circulation (and hence the liver) in a totally different form from that of glucose, *fructose* is the major culprit in the genesis of obesity. What, however, is the evidence for that? In the 1960s he undertook a series of *clinical* investigations which confirmed this, but that evidence has been largely ignored and/or neglected. Assessment of the constituents of systemic capillary or venous blood does *not* necessarily reflect the actual substances which are absorbed into the portal circulation. With many dietary constituents, a profound change occurs during absorption (*ie,* between ingestion into the alimentary tract and presentation to the liver [hepatic] cells). Sucrose, it should again be recalled, consists of two components – *glucose* and *fructose*. In this chapter therefore, most attention is given to one of these components, *ie, fructose*.

It is of course a relatively straightforward matter to determine the ultimate fate of *fructose* following metabolism in the liver; the monosaccharide can be injected intravenously and subsequent venous/capillary blood samples will reveal the resultant metabolic products. However, to assess the absorption products of ingested *fructose* requires precise information on whether or not it actually exists in the form of *fructose* (or alternatively glucose) when presented to the liver (hepatic) cells following absorption into the portal system. Recording results of *in vitro* work in the *Journal of Clinical Investigation*, White and Landau concluded in 1965:

> ... Conversion of fructose to glucose by *human* intestine has been *assumed,* but never established ...[1]

It was this objective which my investigations were designed to confirm or refute *in vivo*.

John Yudkin (*see* Preface) assembled a great deal of *epidemiological data* – accompanied by anecdotal evidence – for an association between excessive '*refined-sugar*' intake, and disease of various organs and systems, much relating to atherosclerosis, and a relationship with myocardial disease, type-2-diabetes mellitus and various intestinal diseases; although he did allude to *obesity*, this was *not* of prime interest. His major thrust was targeted at '*refined-sugar*'s high *calorific* value and of accompanying lack of essential nutrients, portrayed on a backdrop of it being a 'foreign' nutrient – having largely replaced starch – for mammalia in an evolutionary context. There is, however, little in his writing (apart from an excess of calories) to provide a *mechanism* behind the relationship between '*refined-sugar*' intake and disease, or indeed on sucrose absorption and metabolism, although in the context of 'coronary heart disease' he did mention triglycerides.

This chapter seeks to reveal the actual *absorption products* and also the metabolic sequelae of sucrose following ingestion in *H sapiens*. Matt Ridley wrote in an article dated 11 April 2016 – in the context of a *causative* role for *fructose* in obesity – 'Do we know for sure that *fructose* is especially bad? No'. This chapter is also largely an attempt at rebuttal of that statement, and then confirmation that *fructose* is absorbed in man in an entirely different way to that of glucose.[2]

There is evidence that absorption products of sucrose differ in various mammalian species. In the mouse, most *fructose* is altered to glucose during passage across the small-intestinal mucosa, whilst in the rat, most is absorbed in the form of its separate monosaccharides (glucose + *fructose*) molecules. In order to investigate the situation in *H sapiens*, I employed volunteers with a *portal-systemic anastomosis* (PCA), which usually, but not always, arises after a surgical operation seeking to reduce raised portal pressure by short-circuiting the liver. Therefore, by sampling *systemic* blood, absorption products of sucrose following passage across the small-intestinal cells can be *directly* assessed, hepatic *metabolism* being avoided. The result is that absorption products of sucrose can be directly studied. These *clinical* investigations were undertaken at the *Royal Free Hospital* (RFH), London in the 1960s, *ie,* several decades *before* other hypotheses (*see* Chapters 4 and 9) were enunciated, which by no means negate these findings of 50 to 60 years ago!

Absorption products of sucrose in H sapiens

Sucrose and maltose (derived from starch) are now the major dietary saccharides ingested by adult *H sapiens*; 'third World' populations like 'westerners', are now ingesting more sucrose on average than maltose. Very few studies have compared absorption products of these saccharides with those of their constituent monosaccharides in man *in vivo,* most evidence being based on small-intestinal luminal concentrations during intestinal perfusions rather than direct assessment of absorption products. *Fructose* is rarely ingested as a monosaccharide, but as a moiety of sucrose. Whether raised concentration of the separate monosaccharides influences metabolism of the other following intestinal absorption was also unclear in man *in vivo*. In order to determine the situation in man the following *in vivo* investigations in unanaethetised *H sapiens* were thus carried out:

Absorption of sucrose and its constituent monosaccharides

In the first series of investigations, constant intrajejunal (IJ) infusions of sucrose, or of glucose + *fructose* (*ie*, the components of sucrose) took place in *six* patients with cirrhosis (and impaired liver function), and *six* with either a surgical *porta-caval anastomoses* (PCA)[¶¶] or a naturally formed one. To investigate the subsequent fate of *fructose* + glucose when given independently, two further groups consisting of *four* patients in each, with *normal* liver function were given constant intravenous (IV) infusions of either (i) glucose + *fructose*, or *fructose*, or (ii) glucose + *fructose*, or glucose.

The solutions for the intrajejunal (IJ) infusions contained either 292 m-mol 1^{-1} sucrose, 277 m-mol *fructose* + 277m-mol glucose 1^{-1}, 555 m-mol/l *fructose*, or 555 m-mol/l glucose. The intravenous (IV) solutions contained 555 m-mol *fructose* + 555 m-mol glucose 1^{-1}, 555 m-mol 1^{-1} *fructose*, or 555 m-mol 1^{-1} glucose. Each IJ and IV solution was infused at 6.0 ml kg^{-1} hr^{-1} for three hours.

¶¶ In these two groups, small-intestinal blood in effect 'bypasses' the liver (the major 'powerhouse' which *metabolises* food constituents – including the two products of 'refined-sugar'. Therefore dietary constituents appear in capillary and venous blood in the form in which they are presented to the liver cells (hepatocytes).

The *result* indicated that during IJ infusions, blood concentrations of *fructose*, glucose, insulin, pyruvate, lactate and triglyceride-glycerol were similar with both solutions, but in most were mildly higher during sucrose compared with glucose + *fructose* infusions. These minor differences are easily explained by minimal variations in quantities of the monosaccharides during the infusions. Blood concentrations of *fructose*, glucose, insulin, pyruvate and lactate during the IV infusions were *not* influenced by presence of the other monosaccharide (*see* fig 8.1).

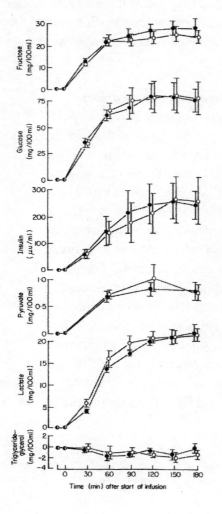

Fig 8.1: Blood concentrations of fructose, glucose, insulin, pyruvate, lactate and trigyceride-glycerol in *six* cirrhotic subjects with either a surgical or spontaneous *portal-systemic anastomosis* (PCA) during *intrajejunal* (IJ) infusions of sucrose (●) and *fructose* + glucose (O) (*see* ref 3).

The *conclusion* was that the findings are entirely consistent with the postulate that *in vivo* in *H sapiens* constituent monosaccharides of sucrose (*ie,,* *fructose* and glucose) are handled by the small intestine along entirely *separate pathways*.[3] They each therefore enter the portal circulation in their (unaltered) original form(s).

Absorption products of the fructose *moiety of sucrose*
In order to determine the fate of *fructose* itself during absorption, the following investigation was undertaken in man *in vivo*. *Fructose* was infused at a constant rate to patients with either normal liver function, cirrhosis, or cirrhosis + PSA, by both intrajejunal (IJ) and intravenous (IV) routes in order to obtain information on absorption products of *fructose* in unanaesthetised man:

> a *fructose* solution (100g 1^{-1}) was infused by IJ and IV routes at a constant mean rate to *six* patients *without* liver disease ('normal' group), *four* with cirrhosis, and *four* with cirrhosis + PSA. Infusions were continued for two hours. Capillary *fructose* concentrations during IJ infusions were significantly higher in the cirrhotic compared with the group with normal liver function. In those with cirrhosis + PSA, concentrations attained during the IJ infusions were up to 85% of those during the IV infusions. Marginally higher capillary *fructose* concentrations were reached in those with cirrhosis during an IV infusion compared with the 'normal' group.
>
> Venous blood lactate tended to attain a slightly higher concentration after both IV and IJ infusions in those with cirrhosis compared with the 'normal' group. In each individual in the group with cirrhosis + PSA, peak lactate concentration was higher during the IJ than IV infusion. Capillary-blood glucose concentrations were higher after both IV and IJ infusions in those with cirrhosis, compared with the 'normal' group. In patients with cirrhosis + PSA, higher peak concentrations were attained during the IJ than IV infusion.
>
> Venous immunoreactive insulin concentration followed that of capillary blood-glucose fairly closely, although the

cirrhotic group without a PSA had a higher concentration compared with other groups during the infusions. It seems likely therefore, that *fructose* – at these infusion rates – does *not* stimulate insulin release, confirming previous observations (*see* figs 8.2 and 8.3).

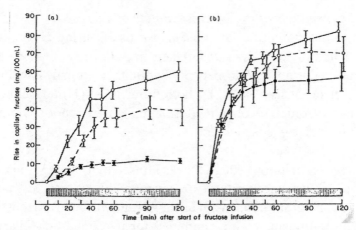

Fig 8.2: Rise in capillary blood *fructose* concentration during intrajejunal (IJ) (left) and intravenous (IV) (right) infusions of *fructose*: ● normal, O - - - O cirrhotic, and O—O cirrhotic + portal-systemic anastomosis (PCA) volunteers (*see* ref 4).

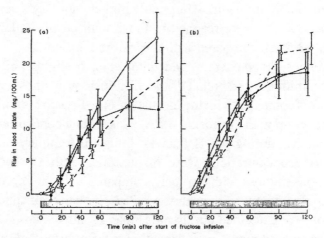

Fig 8.3: Venous-blood lactate concentration in identical individuals to those in fig 8.2 (*see* ref 4) (using similar symbols).

The *conclusion* from this and the previous study is that in *H sapiens*, up to 80–90% *fructose* enters the portal circulation unaltered, while only minor conversion to glucose and lactate occurs. If a metabolite other than *fructose* is produced during absorption, it is clearly to a minute degree.[4]

CONCLUSIONS FROM THESE INVESTIGATIONS

It is therefore clear that most and possibly all, *fructose* presented to the enterocyte brush-border as sucrose is absorbed unchanged, and subsequently metabolised in an entirely different manner to the glucose moiety (the other constituent monosaccharide of sucrose).

Glucose is an essential requirement for life in the *animal* kingdom (not merely in mammals), and is extremely unlikely to exert an injurious effect, apart from over-stimulation of the islets of Langerhans (resulting in *type-2-diabetes mellitus*) even at high concentration – when, for example, ingested as sucrose. In contrast, *fructose*, which is metabolised unaltered in the liver, is both 'foreign' at high concentration to *H sapiens* and probably the entire mammalian kingdom, and does *not* stimulate insulin release, but nevertheless raises blood lactate, pyruvate and triglyceride(s). Therefore, these investigations leave no doubt that following intrajejunal (IJ) administration, nearly all *fructose* is presented to the hepatic cells unaltered. Thus, orally administered *fructose* yields the same metabolites as when given intravenously (IV).

This book has emphasised that *fructose* (a component of sucrose) is now a common dietary component of *H sapiens* throughout the world, and its intake is rapidly increasing. Species variations in absorption products have previously been demonstrated *in vitro* in lower mammals. In one study more lactate was produced in the rat than guinea pig, and up to 30% *fructose* was absorbed as an unidentified compound. Conversion of *fructose* to glucose has also been demonstrated *within* intestinal mucosa of both dog and hamster. In man, *in vitro* evidence for conversion of *fructose* to lactate or glucose *during* absorption has been conflicting, but enzymes for conversion are known to be present in small-intestinal mucosa. One group has shown that up to 70% *fructose* administered *intrajejunally* is converted to glucose *during* absorption, while other investigators have demonstrated minor conversion to lactate but none to glucose, in anaesthetised humans undergoing a surgical operation.

Therefore, assuming that '*refined-sugar*' (sucrose) is a major cause of *obesity*, it is the *fructose* moiety which is clearly likely to be the culprit! More attention should therefore be given to *fructose metabolism* (in the liver) than has formerly been the case![5]

Individual differences in fructose metabolism?

The investigations cited above produced evidence of an individual variation in *fructose* metabolism. It is with that in mind that the following investigation took place. This too was undertaken at the RFH in the 1960s. It was already clear that absorption of *fructose* in *H sapiens* conforms more to the situation in some mammals than others (*see* above). It was also certain that during IV infusion of *fructose* in patients with *normal* liver function, a wide variation in resultant blood lactate concentration exists:

Constant intravenous (IV) (3 h) infusions of a *fructose* solution were given on a rate for body weight basis ($0.6g^{-1}$ kg h^{-1}) to 30 patients *without* evidence of either diabetes mellitus or liver disease. Concentrations of blood *fructose*, pyruvate, lactate and uric acid were monitored, and they formed a plateau during the latter 1–1.5 h of the infusion period. Although numbers were small, individual pyruvate and lactate concentrations at plateau varied greatly, suggesting a bi-modal distribution – indicating two separate groups. That to show a lower pyruvate and lactate rise (group A) contained more males of a mean lower age with ischaemic cardiac disease than the other (group B). Differences were *not* statistically significant – possibly due to relatively small numbers. *Fructose* concentrations at plateau did *not* differ significantly between the groups. Serum *triglyceride-glycerol* concentration during the infusions rose markedly in three patients in group A, but in none in group B. Minor changes to blood glucose, insulin, inorganic phosphate and uric acid concentration *during* the infusions were not significantly different between the groups and did *not* assume a bi-modal distribution.

Constant IV infusions of 0.15m-sodium *lactate* at similar infusion rates and timespan in *eight* (*four* in each group) patients did *not* yield significant differences in blood lactate concentration at plateau in individuals of the two groups (*see* fig 8.4).[6]

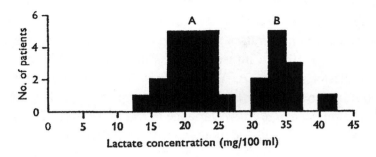

Fig 8.4: Blood-lactate concentration during intravenous (IV) infusions of *fructose*. Groups A contained 19, and B 11 volunteers respectively. Bi-modal distribution in hepatic *fructose* metabolism is suggested (*see* ref 6).

These results therefore clearly reflect qualitative differences in *fructose* metabolism (in the liver) in *H sapiens in vivo*. Variations in *pyruvate* and *lactate* production could be associated with total carbohydrate intake. However, a bi-modal distribution perhaps suggests the possibility of a *genetic* difference in *fructose* metabolism between the groups; more patients would require to be studied for statistical confirmation. Although a bi-modal distribution is not uncommonly demonstrated during drug metabolism, that has *not* been reported with a common dietary constituent. Although relatively large quantities of *fructose* were infused in these investigations, they were not excessive when compared with estimated dietary intake of sucrose by some of the individuals (*see* Chapter 7); *fructose* absorption is in any event highly efficient (*see* above). This investigation also indicates that blood *fructose* concentration reaches a plateau 1.5–2 h after the start of a constant IV infusion, a fact which also applies to blood lactate. At plateau, an equilibrium must inevitably have been reached between *fructose* uptake (from the portal circulation), *metabolism* by the liver, and to a lesser extent adipose tissue.[7]

Lactate clearance after IV infusion of *lactate* is rapid. This was confirmed by continuous infusions which did *not* show a significant difference in *lactate* uptake – *via* pyruvate – between the groups. Differences cannot therefore have resulted from a variation in incorporation of pyruvate into the citric acid cycle. *Lactate* concentration at plateau in each individual bears an approximately linear relationship to weight of *fructose* infused

– previously demonstrated at infusion rates varying from 0.5 to 1.5g kg^{-1} hr^{-1}, using a solution containing 10g 100 ml^{-1}.

Blood lactate concentration *during* the lactate infusions corresponded to approximately 50% of infused *fructose* in circulating blood in group A, and a quarter in group B. Although high blood pryuvate and lactate concentrations are unlikely themselves to be of pathological significance, they clearly reflect a *qualitative* variance in *fructose metabolism* between the groups. It seems likely that more *fructose* was metabolised to pyruvate and lactate by the glycolytic pathway in group B than A, in which a considerable proportion presumably disappeared from the circulation by an alternative pathway. Although differences were *not* statistically significant, rise in serum triglyceride-glycerol concentration *during* the infusions occurred in three patients in group A, possibly associated with greater conversion of *fructose* into α-glycerophosphate and hence to triglyceride in the liver. Relation of patients in this group to those with carbohydrate-induced hyperlipaemia was not investigated.

In *conclusion*, this study suggested two populations with respect to *fructose metabolism*, and could possibly explain differing responses regarding serum triglyceride and uric acid to dietary '*refined-sugar*' (sucrose) in previous studies in *H sapiens*.

POSSIBLE EXPLANATION OF INDIVIDUAL VARIATION IN *FRUCTOSE* METABOLISM

The suggested bi-modal distribution in *fructose metabolism* by hepatocytes, as suggested by this investigation, is consistent with a *genetically* determined difference in concentration of an enzyme involved in *fructose metabolism*. It seems unlikely that *dietary* factors were responsible, but possibly suggest a sex difference between the groups: although those in group A had a higher mean estimated carbohydrate (and sucrose) intake than those in B, some had low, and others in group B a high carbohydrate (and sucrose) intake. Enzyme induction caused by therapeutic agents was *not* responsible, although one patient in each group was consuming a barbiturate at the time of investigation. Differences in either *fructokinase* or liver *fructose-1-phosphate aldolase* between the groups seems unlikely. In *essential benign fructosuria,* in which *fructokinase* is deficient, blood pyruvate and lactate concentrations change marginally after *fructose* ingestion, but blood concentrations of *fructose* are higher than normal, whereas in *hereditary fructose intolerance*, in which *fructose-1-phosphate aldolase* is deficient, abnormally high blood *fructose* concentrations are attained, and hypoglycaemia occurs after oral *fructose*.[8] This result could however, be explained by differing concentrations of an enzyme distal in the *fructose* metabolic pathway. The study incidentally confirms that relatively small amounts of unaltered infused *fructose* are excreted in urine; at the rate used, this amounted to about 2%. Zőllner and his colleagues demonstrated that this was virtually constant after the first 120 min of *fructose* infusion, and they doubted existence of a renal threshold.[9] Fig 8.5 shows a letter from the late Sir Hans Krebs relevant to these results.

METABOLIC RESEARCH LABORATORY

From
H. A. Krebs

NUFFIELD DEPARTMENT OF CLINICAL MEDICINE

Radcliffe Infirmary,
Oxford.

Tel. Oxford 49891, Ext. 244

OX2 6HE

25th February, 1969.

Dr. G.C. Cook,
Department of Medicine,
The Royal Free Hospital,
Gray's Inn Road,
London, W.C.1.

Dear Dr. Cook,

I am afraid I cannot offer really useful comments on your preliminary data on fructose metabolism in man. Similar work has been carried out in several centres (see for example Tygstrup et al., J.Clin.Invest. 47, 817, 1967; Heinz et al., J.Clin.Invest. 47, 1826, 1968; Zalatis & Oliver, Biochem.J. 107, 753, 1967; Zőllner, Klin.Woch., 46, 1300, 1968). However the suggestion that there may be two different kinds of population is certainly new and interesting. It is not likely that there are two major pathways of fructose metabolism. It seems to be more probable that the differences which you notice are due to quantitative variations.

It is certainly possible to assay the key enzymes of fructose metabolism on human liver biopsy specimens. My colleague, L.V. Eggleston, has recently carried out such assays on rat liver samples. He used relatively large quantities of tissue but I believe the methods could be adapted to smaller samples. Should you be interested in these assays I should be glad to supply full particulars. Most of the necessary information is contained, or referred to, in the publications mentioned above.

Yours sincerely,

H.A. Krebs.

Fig 8.5: Comments by Sir Hans Krebs, FRS (1900-81) on the results shown in fig 8.4

Concentrations of blood glucose and insulin during the IV *fructose* infusions were similar to those reported in previous investigations; Zőllner *et al* indicated that IV *fructose* usually produces an initial rise in glucose, independent of infusion rate. In that investigation, infusion rates of 1.0–1.5, but not 0.5 g kg h^{-1} produced subsequent reduction in glucose concentration by around 6 mg 100 ml^{-1} below the fasting concentration. Serum inorganic phosphate concentration fell marginally during the infusions in both groups and were similar to those previously reported. Rise in blood uric acid concentration was lower than previously reported.[10]

Relevance of these findings to recent investigations
Evidence that *fructose* at high concentration is the *cause* of *obesity* has recently been suspected. While *fructose* raises *ghrelin* concentration – which increases hunger (*see* Chapter 9) – it has only limited effect on *leptin* production – responsible for satiety. *Fructose* thus has little or no effect on food satisfaction, but instead *increases* hunger and gluttony – leading to *obesity*; it remains however unclear which *fructose* metabolite stimulates *ghrelin* release.[11] Furthermore, there is now excellent evidence from both animal and human studies that *fructose* metabolism raises blood triglyceride. The investigations cited in this chapter were instigated with arterial disease and *not obesity* as the focus; however, a suggested bi-modal distribution concerning *fructose metabolism* (*see* above) is of interest, it being common knowledge that while some individuals remain slim after ingestion of an excess of '*refined-sugar*', others rapidly become obese. Evidence published in *Proceedings of the National Academy of Sciences* to some extent confirms the results of these studies carried out in the 1960s, and furthermore indicates that *fructose* is handled in the *human* body in a totally different manner to that of glucose; it is both absorbed and metabolised separately, and does *not* stimulate insulin-release. Because insulin promotes appetite diminution and renders food less appealing, ingestion of excessive amounts of *fructose* is undoubtedly an important *cause* of obesity.[1] Journalistic reviews by Taubes have concentrated on current concepts of 'energy balance' (or imbalance), and endocrine hypotheses to account for the present *obesity* pandemic. Those articles however ignore the possibility of a dietary component 'foreign' to the mammalian kingdom. It is perhaps time therefore for current research

to focus on variation in *fructose* metabolism to account for the *obesity* crisis; while some individuals can possibly ingest sucrose with impunity, others are prone to *obesity*.[13]

'*Refined-sugar*' (sucrose) (ingested at *high concentration*), as repeatedly stressed in this book, is historically alien to *H sapiens* and other mammals, although *moderate* quantities of *fructose* in a day-to-day diet have probably existed since time immemorial. *Fructose,* whether presented to the hepatocyte in its mono- or disaccharide form, does *not* stimulate insulin release, but raises blood concentrations of both lactate and pyruvate.[14] It influences triglyceride deposition in both liver and adipose tissue, and also raises uric acid concentrations which would of course account for the recent increase in gout (*see* Chapter 11). The evolutionary hypothesis outlined in Chapter 4 thus becomes increasingly relevant.[15]

Summary and conclusions

The two monosaccharides contained in sucrose are absorbed largely unaltered in *H sapiens*. The human small intestine is therefore unlike that of several other mammals (in which most *fructose* is converted to glucose *during* absorption).[16]

Most investigators have based health hazards of '*refined-sugar*' (sucrose) on *total calories; it* is not easy to understand why the fate of individual *absorption products* of sucrose has hitherto been relatively neglected in this context! Thorough investigation of health hazards of *metabolic* products of highly concentrated sucrose (or *fructose*) intake is urgently required.[17] This chapter might seem both 'academic' and erudite, but is intended to 'unmask' a grossly under-investigated dietary *cause* of human obesity. Effect of a high dietary *fructose* intake on deposition of adipose tissue accompanied by subsequent body weight increase, should be urgently investigated. Its influence on *uric acid* concentration (and gout) also requires further attention.

References and notes

1 L W White, B R Landau. Sugar Transport and Fructose Metabolism in Human Intestine *In vitro. J clin Invest* 1965; 44: 1200–13.

2 J Yudkin. *Pure, white and deadly: how sugar is killing us and what we can do to stop it.* London: Penguin Books 1986: 200; M Ridley. Muddled messages over obesity help nobody: the less fat, more carbohydrate diet was discredited years ago. It makes no sense and should not be public health policy. *Times, Lond* 2016; April 11: 23..

3 G C Cook. Comparison of the absorption and metabolic products of sucrose and its monosaccharides in man. *Clin Sci* 1970; 38: 687–97.

4 G C Cook. Absorption products of D(-) fructose in man. *Ibid* 1969; 37: 675–87.

5 Op cit. *See* notes 3 and 4 above.

6 G C Cook, J Jacobson. Individual variation in fructose metabolism in man. *Br J Nutr* 1971; 26: 187–95.

7 *Ibid.*

8 E R Froesch. In: J B Stanbury, J B Wyngaarden, D S Fredrickson (eds). *The Metabolic Basis of Inherited Disease.* New York: McGraw-Hill 1966: 124.

9 N Zőllner, P K Heuckenkamp, W Nechwatal. *Klin Wshr* 1968; 46: 1300. (*See also*: N Zölner. Eine einfache Modifikation der enzymatischen Harnsaurebestimmung – Normalwerte in der deutschen Bevolkerung. *Z Klin Chem* 1963; 1: 178–82.)

10 *Ibid.*

11 T O'Callaghan. Sickly sweet. *New Scientist* 2014; February 1: 34–9; S Trotter. Fructose effect. *Ibid* 2014; 15 February: 34.

12 O Moody. Obesity clue found in fruit sugar that makes us carry on eating. *Times, Lond* 2015; May 5: 19; S Luo, J R Monterosso, K Sarpelleh, K A Page. Differential effects of fructose versus glucose on brain and appetite responses to food cues and decisions for food rewards. *Proc Nat Acad Sci USA* 2015; 12: 3020–6. (*See also*: note 9 above.)

13 G Taubes. The Science of obesity: what do we really know about what makes us fat? *Br med J* 2013; 346: 16–19; G Taubes. *The Case against Sugar* London; Portobello Books 2017: 365.

14 Op cit. *See* note 2 above. (*See also*: G C Cook. Absorption and

metabolism of D(-) fructose in man. *Am J clin Nutr* 1971; 234: 1302–7.)

15 J Leake. Obesity epidemic linked to chubby chimp gene. *Sunday Times, Lond* 2015; November 15: 27. (*See also* Chapter 4.)

16 Op cit. *see* note 1 above.

17 Anonymous. High fructose corn syrup. *Br med J* 2015; October 31: 3.

CHAPTER 9:

Appetite-associated hormones: *leptin* and *ghrelin*

In theory, physiological (*ie,* hormonal) mechanisms underlying appetite regulation should be effective in regulation of body weight. In practice, according to research at the *University of Sheffield* and published in *Critical Reviews in Food Science and Nutrition*, 'feeling full' doesn't though stop excessive eating! In this short chapter, therefore, the rôle, and limitation of two neuropeptide hormones is addressed.[1] Discovery of these hormones has encouraged research in this area, but has limited work on constituents of '*refined-sugar*' themselves.

The two hormones involved in weight-maintenance are: *ghrelin* and *leptin*; ideally their joint function creates weight homeostasis. The term *leptin* is derived from a Greek word λεhoc (or leptos) meaning thin – the *satiety* hormone; *ghrelin* is derived from proto-Indo-European languages indicating *grow. Ghrelin*, too, is a peptide hormone, which is also known as lenomoreline – the *hunger* hormone. Both are active in controlling appetite, which is accomplished by influencing *hypothalamic* function. Although between them, weight-constancy would be anticipated, there is a significant flaw in this simplistic view of events. *Leptin* resistance (comparable to insulin-resistance) frequently results, and a vicious cycle consequently ensues:

- Increased appetite leads to increased fat and obesity,
- Increased fat stimulates greater *leptin* output,
- Excessive fat also disrupts *leptin* signalling,
- The *hypothalamus* senses starvation, with *increased* (instead of decreased) appetite, and
- *Increase* in appetite is associated with further weight-*gain* and increased *obesity.*

Leptin *(the 'appetite hormone')*
Leptin is produced by adipose cells as well as in other sites, and regulates energy balance by inhibiting hunger. In obesity, decreased sensitivity to *leptin* results in inability to detect *satiety* despite high energy stores.

The discovery of *leptin* (first of the appetite hormones to be documented) – secreted by adipose tissue – is as follows. The saga began with experimental work by D L Coleman (1931–2014)[2] at Maine, Germany in the 1960s and 70s. He was working on two overweight *mouse* models: *ob* (obese) and *db* (diabetic) strains, which had been recognised since 1951 and 54, respectively. A series of experiments demonstrated that blood from a *normal* mouse caused weight-loss in the *ob* strain. Also, blood from the *db* mouse caused the *normal* one to starve to death. Thus, in obesity a hormonal factor seemed almost certain. In the 1990s, Jeffrey Friedman (1954–present), of Rockefeller University, USA, actually identified this appetite-suppressing hormone – *leptin*. In humans, however, obesity is more likely to be associated with *leptin*-resistance – (*see* above) (comparable to insulin-resistance in *type-2-diabetes mellitus*). Secretion does *not* seem to be affected by presence of dietary *fructose*.[3]

The structure of *leptin* was unravelled in 1994; it does indeed suppress appetite, thus enhancing satiety, concentration being lower in thin compared with obese individuals. Many obese individuals however, have developed resistance to these suppressive effects (*see* above). Although secreted primarily by fat cells (*see* above), it is also produced by the stomach, heart, pancreas, placenta, and skeletal muscle. *Leptin* thus *reduces* appetite, and when an increase in dietary fat occurs, the higher is the resulting concentration of this hormone.

A therapeutic agent, semaglutide, with a similar action to *leptin* in diminishing appetite is currently undergoing *clinical* trials at Leeds and Leicester.[4]

Ghrelin *(lenomorelin) (the 'hunger hormone')*
This neuropeptide was discovered in 1999 by M Kojima and colleagues, and is secreted by ghrelinergic cells in the stomach, duodenum, jejunum, pancreatic islets and other sites in the gastrointestinal tract. *Ghrelin* is secreted by an empty stomach and, like *leptin*, acts on the *hypothalamus* – where it both *increases* appetite in response to hunger, stimulating

gastric acid secretion, and has a significant rôle in regulating distribution rate and use of energy. When the stomach is distended, secretion ceases. Overall therefore, it promotes hunger, gastric acid secretion and hence preparation for food intake. The cerebral receptor is identical to that of *leptin* (also designated the '*satiety* hormone') – which has an opposing effect.

This hormone thus functions as an adiposity signal between the brain and the body's energy store(s). With weight-loss, *ghrelin* concentration *increases*, thus producing a rise in food consumption with the result that weight increases; after this occurs however, concentration of the hormone decreases, with an accompanying *decrease* in both food consumption and weight-loss. Overall, therefore, *ghrelin* acts as a body-weight regulator, its major rôle being a reverse of that of *leptin*. As well as regulating hunger however, *ghrelin* plays a significant part in energy homeostasis; incidentally, it also has a rôle in promoting sexual desire and in development of various addictions.

Normally, if an individual is under-eating, *ghrelin* concentration increases, but in the event of over-eating it usually decreases. However, in children who are both obese and consuming 'fizzy drinks' between meals, instead of switching off (which it normally does for some three hours *after* a meal) it remains constantly low.[5]

Importance of these two hormones in weight-maintenance?
It is so far unknown to what extent precisely these two hormones play in weight-homeostasis. Some (mostly German) researchers claim that they are absolutely critical, while others are far more sceptical.

Hormone concentrations in sleep deprivation
In sleep deficiency, it is now known that **leptin** concentration falls, while that of **ghrelin** rises. This results in an *increase* in appetite, involving '*refined-sugar*' in particular. These events might thus be especially important in children in whom sleep-lack is now common.[6]

Surgical implications
Gastric bypass surgery (*see* Chapter 15) reduces both capacity for food within the gastro-intestinal tract, and also reduces *ghrelin* concentration

in comparison with lean controls, and those with dietary-controlled weight-loss. Vertical sleeve gastrectomy also reduces plasma *ghrelin* concentration by up to 60%. *Ghrelin* is also suspected, but not proved, to enhance both pancreatic and other forms of gastrointestinal malignancy.

Other cerebral centres with a rôle in weight-control
The major *cause* in a minority of cases of obesity is to be found in the brain. In a study carried out at the *Montreal Neurological Institute and Hospital* which was published in *Psychological Science* it was shown that with awareness of the calorific content of various items of food, areas of the brain – already known to be implicated in evaluation of food options – were influenced. Greater understanding of these might perhaps lead to control of those factors resulting in obesity.[7] *Asprosin* is a newly discovered hormone which is released by fat cells, in turn stimulating hepatocytes (liver cells) to release glucose into the circulation; with this rise, hormonal release is 'switched-off'. Individuals with *neotnatal progeroid syndrome* however, lack this mechanism and in consequence are thin. If release of this hormone could be blocked, obesity and *type-2-diabetes* would, in theory, be prevented.[8]

Research at *Macquarie University, Australia*, has indicated that a diet high in both fat and '*refined-sugar*' encourages increased 'snacking' after a meal; this is probably also mediated *via* the *hypothalamus*.[9]

Experimental studies
A recent article in the *Journal of Endocrinology* is of interest in the context of weight-reduction. A report from *Oregon State University* and the *University of Florida* concentrated on work in adult female rats. Intra-cerebral injections of a gene stimulating *leptin* production resulted in significant weight-loss. This was caused by appetite-suppression, which the researchers considered more effective than dieting. It was devoid of triggering osteoporosis – a common side-effect of *diet*-induced weight-loss. It will clearly be many years however, before such a procedure could possibly be applicable in *Homo sapiens*.[10]

An investigation on mice at the *Yale School of Medicine,* published in *The Journal of Clinical Investigation*, has indicated that by blocking a 'small nuclear receptor' (responsible for production of a protein which prevents hunger) in the *hypothalamus*, obesity has been avoided, despite ingestion of a diet high in both sugar and fat. If applicable to *H sapiens*, this might assist in prevention of both obesity and also *type 2 diabetes*.[11]

Conclusion(s)

It is clear that *gut-hormones* have a significant rôle in weight-homeostasis. It is though relatively early to evaluate their place in regulation of obesity.

Perhaps opinion is swinging back to the 1930s and *obesity* is after all, in part a 'glandular' (*ie,* hormonal) disorder! In the meantime it is important to carefully re-assess present knowledge and in particular, the part played by the *fructose* component of sucrose in this saga. In any case, a 'sugar tax' should be introduced, even though the future rôle of hormone control of appetite remains unpredictable.[12]

References and notes

1   T Whipple. Feeling full does not stop you eating more. *Times, Lond* 2016; October 19: 23. (*see also*: J Wass. Obesity action plan. *Ibid* 2017; September 6: 28).

2   Anonymous. Professor Douglas Coleman: geneticist who discovered that obesity could be linked to hormones. *Ibid* 2014: May 26: 49.

3   T O'Callaghan. Sickly sweet. *New Scientist* 2014; February 1: 34–9.

4   O Moody. Drug promises top speed up battle against obesity. *Times, Lond* 2017; October 24: 6.

5   B Perry, Y Wang. Appetite regulation and weight control: the role of gut hormones. *Nutrition and Diabetes*. 2012; 2: 26. (*See also*: R M Nass, D B Gaylinn, A D Rogol, M O Thorner. Ghrelin and growth hormone: the story in reverse. *Proc N Acad Sci* 2010; 107: 8501–2.)

6   M Walker. *Why We Sleep: the new science of sleep and dreams*. London: Allan Lane 2017: 171–8; T Whipple. Sweet dreams: a good night's sleep helps you to cut sugar. *Times, Lond* 2018; January 10: 22.

7   Anonymous. Sweets on the brain? Blame your internal calorie counter. *Ibid* 2014; October 21: 15.

8   Anonymous. 'Thin' hormone could fight diabetes and obesity. *New Scientist* 2016; April 23: 16.

9   K Lay. Hormone jab beats dieting for weight-loss. *Times, Lond* October 21: 18. (*see also*: O Moody. Drug promises to speed up battle against obesity. *Ibid* 2017: 6.)

10 S Hazel. Why sweet and fatty foods make us keep eating. *Ibid* 2016; July 13: 14.

11 K Burgess. How to eat what you want and still stay slim (the secret is in your brain). *Ibid* 2014; August 2: 16.

12 F Field. Sugar and hunger. *Ibid* 2015; October 23: 32.

Chapter 10:

Dental complications of 'refined-sugar'

This chapter has little to do with obesity, but much about a consequence of ingesting one of its major causes – the dietary component '*refined-sugar*' (sucrose). Possessing a 'sweet tooth', although an underlying *cause* of obesity, has of course little to do with dental status but much to do with a craving for *sweetness*! Nevertheless, the *first* thought that the *effect* of '*refined-sugar*' on human (and other mammals) health arouses is probably directed to dental caries and *not* obesity.

Britons consume more than twice as much sugar in a day than the ideal. An association between caries and '*refined-sugar*' content of food has been known for many centuries (*see* below), which was emphasised yet again in the correspondence columns of the London *Times* newspaper in 2014.[1] Influence of '*refined-sugar*' (sucrose) on teeth has been the substance of numerous books and several recent articles, a sucrose-rich environment favouring growth of *Streptococcus mutans, Str sobrinus* and *Lactobacillus* sp. These acid-producing bacteria attack both enamel and dentine; sucrose has the property of producing dextran which serves as an ideal substrate for survival of relevant bacteria. A genetic factor is also undoubtedly involved, but there is no doubt that fluoride in toothpaste and drinking water is in part protective. *Caries* (derived from the Latin word 'rottenness') are also associated with socio-economic status, lower classes being particularly vulnerable.

John Yudkin, writing in the 1960s, strongly opposed to excessive dietary '*refined-sugar*', referred to a steep *decline* in childhood dental caries in the previous decade – probably, he felt, due principally to fluoridisation of drinking water and toothpaste, rather than a reduction in '*refined-sugar*' intake! However, in developing countries, with a steep rise in '*refined-sugar*' consumption, the situation is rapidly deteriorating. He also referred to a reduction in dental caries during the two world wars (1914–18 and 1939–45) when 'sugar was scarce'; but, like most of his conclusions, these were mere *associations* rather than 'cause effect' relationships. He concluded nevertheless by suggesting that 'sticky sweets, cakes and biscuits *between* meals are major culprits …' because these substances stick to the teeth; taking a snack *between* meals is also bad for teeth.

Britain apparently has the worst rate of tooth decay in western Europe. Sparkling water and lager (the arbitrary risk factors of 0.1 and 0.6 respectively) are of minor importance as far as enamel erosion is concerned; *cola* (0.7) and white wine (2.2) are considered moderate, but apple (4.5) and grapefruit (9.3) juices present a high risk. It is recommended that these drinks if consumed at all, should be taken *with* meals and *not* as snacks *between* them.[2]

In *hereditary fructose intolerance,* which Yudkin also cited in his book, ingestion of either *fructose* or sucrose produce nausea and vomiting, resulting in elimination of these sugars from diets in early life. Sufferers from this *rare* inherited disease therefore ingest 'starchy foods' instead, and as a result prevalence of caries is negligible.

Writing about the present state of children's teeth, described as a 'national disgrace' and undoubtedly associated with '*refined-sugar*', a correspondent from Scotland has affirmed this fact.[3]

Historical incidence of caries
Yudkin claimed that fossil evidence indicated that dental caries 'hardly existed in prehistoric times' and that this disease has only recently become far more common. Although in fact, physical anthropologists have long considered that human tooth decay did not arise until some 10,000 years ago, when farming, ingestion of carbohydrates, and encouragement of 'sugar-loving' bacteria began, recent evidence is not altogether consistent with this fact. There is proof that dental caries began to afflict *Homo sapiens* a *very* long time ago. It is perhaps pertinent to stress that although dinosaurs developed teeth which 'could tear through bone and sinew', *Australopithecus* (three or four million years ago) was to some extent affected by *caries*.[4] Neanderthals, some 50,000 years ago, were perhaps 'early adopters of a five-a-day diet', and dietary intake, according to fossilised evidence from Spain, consisted of 'a mix of vegetables, berries and nuts' (*see* Chapter 7). However, diet was then 'dominated by meat', constituting the first clear evidence that primates 'enjoyed an omnivorous

diet' – since then, survival advantage for hominins has of course devolved around *improved nutrition*.[5] The diet of a Palaeolithic caveman has been outlined in a graphic account published in 2014 (*see also* Chapter 7).[6] Evidence of filling of caries (using hair and tar) of 13,000-year-old teeth in northern Italy (*ie,* during the last Ice Age***) has corroborated presence of caries many centuries ago.[7] Another study has produced confirmatory evidence for the *Neolithic* period (4000–2500 BC); a 4,000-year-old burial site in the Scottish highlands (dated at 1982 BC–1889 BC) revealed a woman in her 40's with advanced tooth decay. During the *Neolithic* period, caries were however probably caused by plant foods – which contained large amounts of carbohydrates. An increase of caries in South Asia was probably associated with *rice* consumption. Also, the Ebers Papyrus (c.1550 BC) has mention of 'rotten teeth'. Recently, a late 30-year-old 2,200-year-old mummy in the *National Museum of Israel* has been shown to possess dental caries; his dental state was attributed to 'too much time indoors [coupled with] a diet rich in carbohydrates'.

It is well known that wheat and barley – ground to produce porridge and bread – are considerably higher in 'sugar' than is the case with *wild* fruits and grains, but a transition from a nomadic hunter-gatherer lifestyle to a farming one was probably less clear-cut than formerly maintained! The *Times* newspaper has also focused on Moroccan hunter-gatherers of 13,000 (range 1500 BC–13,700) BC in a pre-agricultural society. Of 52 adult jaws examined at the *Natural History Museum* in London, only three were completely free of dental caries, the cause being considered a diet of acorns and snails, and *not* a result of sucrose; the former, after storage (necessary to counteract seasonal 'food stress') containing a high concentration of carbohydrate, and the latter 'abrasive particles'.

During medieval times, incidence of caries, which had certainly remained low during the bronze (2500 BC–800 BC) and iron (800 BC–AD 43) periods escalated, sugar-cane very slowly becoming available in the western world from about 1000 AD onwards. Interestingly, victims of the Pompeii volcano eruption (AD 79), although most were relatively young, had little evidence of tooth decay.[8] Evidence from archaeological investigations associated with HMS *Mary Rose*, a ship which sank in the Solent during the reign of King Henry VIII (1491–1547), has indicated

---

*** This *Ice Age* existed from 1.8 million to 11,700 years (*ie* the beginning of the *Pleistocene* epoch) ago.

that sailors at that time had 'excellent teeth'.[9] Queen Elizabeth I [1533–1603] at the beginning of her reign in 1558, was apparently importing substantial amounts of 'refined-sugar' from Morocco and other Islamic states; her father, King Henry VIII had encouraged contact(s) with those countries in order to exert a significant impact on the British economy, one estimate being that within a decade, imports of 250 tons/year and worth £18,000 of 'refined-sugar', were made. Some have attributed Elizabeth's *black teeth* to the vast quantities of 'refined-sugar' in her diet.

There seems to have been a marked increase of tooth decay in the early *nineteenth* century – almost certainly diet-related.[10]

PERIODONTAL DISEASE

Another article, quoting one in the *British Dental Journal*, highlighted relative rarity of *periodontal* disease amongst ancient Romans in England. An analysis of three hundred skulls of Roman Britons at Poundbury, Dorset, revealed for example, a relatively low incidence (5–10%) of periodontitis compared with approximately 30% in present-day Britons. The conclusion was that lack of dietary 'refined-sugar', diabetes mellitus and smoking underlay these findings. An accompanying leading article referred to a steady decline in 'oral health during following millennia'.[11]

Prevention of caries

Avoidance of bacteria-loving carbohydrates in a *twenty-first* century diet is clearly 'easier said than done'! A morning cup of coffee is apparently good for the teeth, for it 'breaks down *S mutans* and other bacteria associated with tooth decay', but on the other hand added milk with *sugar* is counter-productive; this conclusion came from a study published in the *Journal of Applied Microbiology* which demonstrated that coffee contains polyphenols, and reduces bacterial adhesiveness, both of which are factors in formation of dental caries.[12] An article in *BMC Public Health* recorded that researchers had indicated that daily 'refined-sugar' intake should be limited to 15 grams – equivalent to 'one can of *cola*'. Tooth decay in a world context, it concluded, paralleled increase in sugar consumption; this article also cited evidence from several overseas countries associating 'refined-sugar' with prevalence of dental caries.[13]

Incidentally, one advantage of artificial sweeteners (*see* Chapter 14) is that they do *not* provide a suitable substrate for *S mutans* and other caries-forming bacteria, and therefore caries are rarely a problem in their use.

Children's teeth

Several articles in London's *Times* and *Sunday Times* newspapers have focused on the state of *children*'s teeth. This is also a serious problem in <5-year-old infants, who frequently require extractions of 'milk teeth'. According to *Public Health England*, in a study of 50,000 children more than one tenth of three-year-olds had evidence of tooth decay, the worst being in: the north-west London, Yorkshire and the Humber regions; this article stressed that it was an entirely *preventable* disease, avoidance of which is dependent on less *'refined-sugar'*, coupled with tooth-brushing using fluoride toothpaste. Also, widespread fluoridation of water-supplies was advocated. The long-standing controversy about fluoride in water supplies has recently re-erupted; although there are significant disadvantages, surely beneficial effect on children's teeth outweighs these. Intake of sugary drinks has been reduced in a *public health* campaign in Liverpool.[14] Once again, manufacturers are targeting children; toothpaste recommended for infants and children costs double the price of the adult product, although ingredients are identical! If children *must* consume 'fizzy drinks', they should be consumed through a straw, thus minimising resultant caries.

Apparently, 26,000 English children of 5–9 years old, *ie,* nearly five hundred weekly, were actually admitted to hospital for multiple tooth extractions during 2013–14; most extractions required a general anaesthetic.[15] Another report, while recording that some 50% of children have tooth decay –blamed on 'sugary drinks' together with lack of tooth brushing – indicated that confidence and 'self-esteem' associated with reluctance to smile was a result.[16]

Obesity and tooth decay

In south Wales, a dental surgeon has issued a letter to the effect that 'anyone heavier than a 20-stone [127 kg] recommended maximum weight' will have to 'find treatment elsewhere' because: (i) dental chairs are *not* designed for obese individuals, and (ii) 'the [dental] staff could injure themselves helping overweight patients in and out of the chairs'.[17]

References and notes

1 O Moody. Sweet-toothed Britain is named and shamed. *Times, Lond* 2016: June 4:4; D Douglas. Sugar fillings. *Ibid* 2014; October 9: 33.

2 J Yudkin. *Pure, White and Deadly: how sugar is killing us and what we can do to stop it.* London: Penguin Books 2012: 127–33; O Moody. Fruit snacking is a rotten idea for your teeth, warn dentists. *Times, Lond* 2015: May 9: 33. (*See also*: note 1 above; C Smyth. Elderly in care homes plagued by tooth decay. *Ibid* 2016; July 5: 21; T Whipple. Sweet tooth? Blame it on hormones. *Ibid* 2017: May 3: 3.)

3 Op cit. *See* notes 1 and 2 above.

4 Anonymous. How T rex munched its way to top of the food chain. *Times, Lond* 2015; July 29: 16.

5 H Devlin. Contains nuts: why Neanderthals took to the 5-a-day diet. *Ibid* 2014; 27 June: 27; A Botelho. Humans had rotten teeth before farming. *New Scientist* 2014; January 11: 13; T Whipple. Why early man needed a toothbrush. *Times, Lond* 2014; January 7: 20; G Carlstrom. The curse of the mummy: tooth rot and brittle bones. *Ibid* 2016; July 29: 35. (*See also*: D Alberge. Bad teeth and a broken nose: meet man from 7,500 BC. *Sunday Times, Lond* 2016; November 20: 12.)

6 H Devlin. Neanderthals used teeth as 'third hand'. *Times, Lond* 2014; June 20: 23; R Crampton. Smoked pigeon and fry-ups? Yes, I'd love to eat like a caveman: in the last 60 years our diet has changed more than in the previous 10,000. Should we eat more like our ancestors? *Times 2, Lond* 2014; November 20: 6–7.

7 P Willan. Ice Age dentist made fillings of hair and tar. *Times, Lond* 2017; April 12: 36.

8 T Kington. For perfect teeth, follow the Pompeii diet. *Ibid* 2015: October 1: 3.

9 Anonymous. Sugar-free diet not enough to stop Bronze Age toothache. *Ibid* 2014; February 14: 20; Anonymous. Margaret Rule: archaeologist who led two of the most dramatic British excavations of the last century – the discovery of the Roman palace at Fishbourne and the raising of the wreck of the Tudor warship, the Mary Rose in the Solent. *Ibid* 2015; April 18: 76–7; V Low. Mary Rose emerges in all her glory: the hull of Henry VIII's flagship is shown for the

first time without the trappings of restoration. *Ibid* 2016: July 20: 13; J Brotton. *This Orient Isle: Elizabethan England and the Islamic World.* London: Allen Lane 2016: 358.

10 *Ibid*

11 T Whipple. Why Romans had teeth to smile about: they may have been decadent but they had less gum disease than 21st century Britons. *Times, Lond* 2014; October 24: 3. (*See also*: Anonymous. Of Ancient Extraction: What did the Romans do for us? Minimise gum disease, of course. *Ibid* 2014; October 24: 36.)

12 H Devlin. Wake up and swill the coffee … then smile. *Ibid* 2014; June 11: 13.

13 K Lay. Call for sugar controls in fight against tooth decay. *Ibid* 2014; September 16: 11.

14 L Bannerman. City targets sugary drinks to curb child tooth decay. *Ibid* 2016; May 9: 19; O Moody. A tenth of children have rotting teeth. *Ibid* 2014; September 30: 23; E Crouch. Fluoride and teeth. *Ibid* 2016; November 2: 26; Baldwin of Bewdley. Tooth and nail fight over fluoride. *Ibid* 2016; November 3: 28; P Langmaid. Benefit of fluoride. *Ibid* 2016; November 5: 30.

15 S-K Templeton. Rotten teeth put 26,000 children in hospital. *Sunday Times, Lond* 2014; July 13: 1; S-K Templeton. Rotten teeth in toddlers at crisis level. *Ibid* 2015; July 12: 1; A Ellson. Child toothpaste is money down the tube. *Times, Lond* 2016; April 16: 9; K Gibbons. Child tooth decay hits record high. *Ibid* 2017; January 11: 14; Anonymous. Toothless: time to wield a big stick against children's relentless consumption of sugar. *Ibid* 2017; January 12: 27; G Newman. Child tooth decay. *Ibid* 2017; January 14: 26; B Scott. Tooth trouble. *Ibid* 2017; January 16: 28; C Smyth. Smile! British teeth are no longer a laughing stock. *Ibid* 2017; March 21: 20.

16 C Smyth. Rotten teeth are secret reason why teens don't smile. *Ibid* 2015; March 20: 17;

17 S de Bruxelles. Dentist turns away patients too fat for the chair. *Ibid* 2015; July 31: 11.

CHAPTER 11:

Systemic complications of excessive 'refined-sugar' ingestion and obesity

This chapter focuses on complications of being either overweight or obese. Dental decay (*see* Chapter 10) is clearly a direct result of an excessive '*refined-sugar*' intake rather than obesity itself. Numerous associated-diseases have been well documented, not least the effects of obesity on weight-bearing joints. However, recent coverage has mostly targeted *five* groups of systemic entities – all of which receive attention in the next few pages:

- Diabetes mellitus (DM) – probably the most frequent complication of obesity. Possibly the greatest importance of this complication to Britain is its cost, which threatens to destroy the *National Health Service* [NHS],
- Hypertension and cardiac disease,
- Gout (probably a result of excessive '*refined-sugar*' (sucrose) rather than a direct result of obesity), and also other arthritides,
- Dementia, and
- Certain malignancies.

John Yudkin recorded several systemic *clinical* complications arising from excessive 'sugar' consumption in the 1960s, but his overwhelming theme was of an *association* with *ischaemic heart disease* rather than obesity. Apart from *dental caries* (*see* Chapter 10), he cited: *type-2-diabetes mellitus*, opthalmic disease, dermatological problems, joint diseases (especially gout), hepatological abnormalities, various digestive disorders, and a possible link with malignancy. He also speculated on interference with the action of certain therapeutic agents.[1]

Diabetes mellitus

It is widely known that obesity carries a significant risk of development of *type-2-diabetes mellitus* (DM). In 2014, the London *Times* newspaper carried a banner headline on its front page: '**One in three now at risk as diabetes levels soar**' (*see* fig 11.1). 'Britain [the article claimed] faces a diabetes "time bomb" …' which could well bankrupt the *National Health Service*. While more than three million people in Britain already have DM, it continued, 'within a decade this could well reach five million'. In 2003, 11.6% of Britain's adults had DM, but by 2011 this had risen to 35.3%, the *speed* of the rise being deemed especially disturbing. The Chief Executive of *Diabetes UK* was reported as saying in 2015 that 'Unless we make people aware of [the] risk of *type-2-diabetes mellitus* [there is a likelihood that] we could see an even greater increase … one tenth of the NHS budget [being] currently devoted to this disease'. The rise in prescriptions for diabetes drugs has increased by 80% in the last decade.[2] A follow-up letter to the article from a British primary-health-care worker confirmed that the disease had already reached *epidemic* proportions.[3]

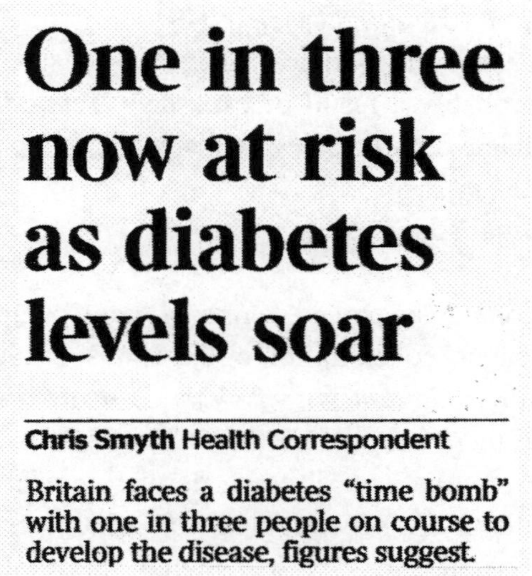

One in three now at risk as diabetes levels soar

Chris Smyth Health Correspondent

Britain faces a diabetes "time bomb" with one in three people on course to develop the disease, figures suggest.

Fig 11.1: Headline to an article in the London *Times* newspaper (2014; June 10: 1–2) recording the vast increase in incidence of *Diabetes mellitus* in Britain.

The magnitude of this obesity-related disease, was once again highlighted in an article published in early 2016, which reported a 'silent explosion' of diabetes worldwide; this, the newspaper emphasised, in an accompanying leading article was now a 'silent killer' which required co-ordinated international action.[4] The fact that overweight or obese children were developing *type-2-diabetes* was also highlighted in mid-2016 – 'with a third of 10-year-olds either overweight or obese in the UK, it has become increasingly common to see children and young people developing *type-2-diabetes*'. Another article stressed that with this explosion of cases of DM, depression and dementia (at present a highly topical subject – *see* below) becomes a serious threat.[5] while a *British Medical Journal* (BMJ) editorial concluded that 'strong evidence points to an association between DM and several major malignancies (colorectal, breast, endometrial, liver, pancreatic, and bladder)' (*see* below).[6]

A study carried out by the *University of Copenhagen* and published in the *Journal of Clinical Endocrinology and Metabolism* indicated (confirming previous suspicions) that 'heavy use' of antibiotics, by altering the spectrum of colonic bacteria, might predispose to *type-2-diabetes mellitus*.[7] Meanwhile, several articles tackled strategies to *prevent*, *control* and *manage type-2-diabetes mellitus* (*see* below).[8]

A somewhat controversial article dealt with obesity, diabetics and mortality! A significant risk of DM as a complication of obesity in previously fit young individuals is especially relevant in those with a family history of the disease, and in certain ethnic groups, including: South Asians, Black Africans and those with an African-Caribbean origin.[9]

PREVENTION

Various strategies have been suggested to deal with the problem! Concentration on weight reduction has obviously been stressed.[10] Most emphasis has been given to diet – beginning with efforts to encourage breast-feeding.[11] But, what *specific* items of diet are likely to be beneficial? And is the timing of meals important? Several attempts have been made to answer these questions.[12]

On a more encouraging note, another article referred to research published in *BMC Medicine* indicating that daily yoghurt (but *not* other dairy products) ingestion might reduce the risk of DM, the protective effect probably resulting from bacterial content of yoghurt, or possibly its calcium and/or magnesium content. Other positive factors cited in prevention were: a daily glass of red wine, and/or (surprisingly perhaps) pre-existent hypercholesterolaemia.[13]

A study published in *Annals of Internal Medicine*, based on a follow-up of 10,500 people at Kingston-upon-Hull over ten years (the precise causes of death was *not* recorded) demonstrated that overweight individuals suffering from *type-2-diabetes* live longer than those who are either of normal weight or those who are underweight. This paradoxical finding might of course have an alternative explanation, *eg*, those of normal or sub-normal weight might smoke and/or drink more![14]

TREATMENT

A concise summary of the *National Institute for Health and Care Excellence* (NICE) recommendations for sufferers from *type-2-diabetes* was assembled in the *BMJ* for 2016.[15] What though is the rôle of bariatric surgery? While there is some evidence that the disease can be *cured* by this method, another article indicated that weight-loss surgery was currently being denied to otherwise suitable patients by the *National Health Service*.[16]

Humans are however apparently not alone in suffering from this increase in DM; the *Sunday Times* related that overfed *cats* also suffer from the disease, and a 'diabetes clinic' has recently been opened to care for them. Average weight of cats has incidentally increased by 25%, and their likelihood of developing DM is four times higher than thirty years previously.[17]

Hypertension, cardiac disease and stroke

In addition to a list of well-established complications of obesity, as well as excessive '*refined-sugar*' intake, a recent article added hypertension and related heart disease, especially in children (*see* fig 11.2) (*see also* Chapter 3). A report in the *American Journal of Clinical Nutrition* recorded an excellent correlation between '*refined-sugar*' ingestion and hypertension.[18]

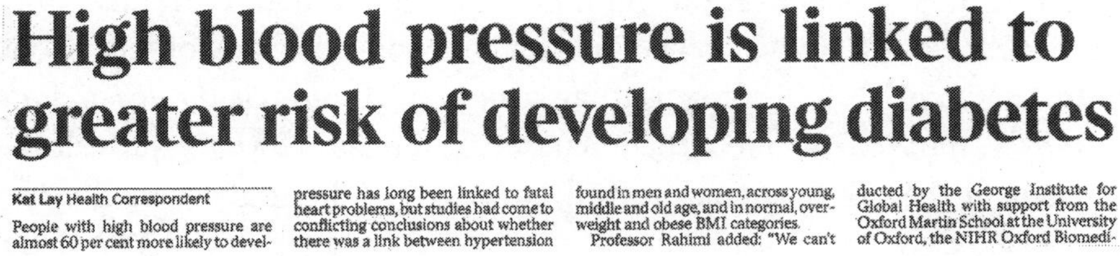

High blood pressure is linked to greater risk of developing diabetes

Kat Lay Health Correspondent

People with high blood pressure are almost 60 per cent more likely to devel- pressure has long been linked to fatal heart problems, but studies had come to conflicting conclusions about whether there was a link between hypertension found in men and women, across young, middle and old age, and in normal, over- weight and obese BMI categories. Professor Rahimi added: "We can't ducted by the George Institute for Global Health with support from the Oxford Martin School at the University of Oxford, the NIHR Oxford Biomedi-

Fig 11.2: Headline in the London *Times* newspaper (2015; September 29: 17) emphasising the association between DM and hypertension.

This association between *'refined-sugar'* intake and hypertension – a known cause of heart attacks (myocardial infarction) – has recently been confirmed; association with diet had previously involved *salt* and hypertension, but an article in the *American Journal of Cardiology* claimed that this link was misguided. The *conclusion* from that important article is that the *fructose* component of the sucrose molecule increases blood pressure 'in a manner [totally] independent of *sodium* intake'[19], a fact that has also been highlighted elsewhere.[20]

Interestingly, a study also in the *Journal of The American College of Cardiology* indicated that hypertension and stroke (in some cases resulting from excessive *'refined-sugar'* consumption) poses in itself a risk factor to subsequent development of diabetes (*see* above).[21]

Although an alarming rise in prevalence of cerebro-vascular accident (stroke) in relatively young individuals – aged 40–50 years – was reported in 2015, this has since been shown to be largely due to *undiagnosed* hypertension coupled with lack of exercise. The influence of *obesity* in this association should however not be underestimated.[22]

Gout and other arthritides (including osteo-arthritis)
Britain, in view of its high frequency of obesity, is heading for an 'arthritis epidemic', warned *Arthritis Research UK* in 2014; the 'pernicious myth' that exercise is bad for joints must, it stressed, be put to rest! Obese individuals are 'up to six times as likely to develop osteoarthritis compared with those whose weight is normal'. In one study, in a group of obese women a loss of 5kg *halved* the risk of arthritis; furthermore, the article claimed 'activity can help to *cure* the condition'.[23]

It is estimated that over one million British individuals currently suffer from *gout*, and a rise of 64% has, for example, been recorded at one hospital since 1997. Referring to an article in *Annals of the Rheumatic Diseases*, the *BMJ* also recorded that during the last 15 years, prevalence of gout in the UK has soared, and is presently the highest in Europe. However, only one third – one in 40 – of individuals (*ie, 2.5%* of the population) affected was receiving a urate-lowering drug.[24] In two articles emphasising re-emergence of this *historical* disease (*see* fig 11.3) in the last decade, the *Times* listed several famous individuals who suffered from the ailment:

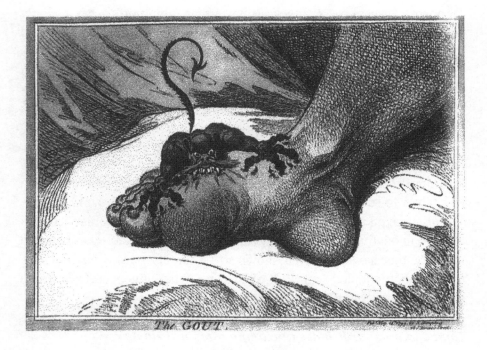

Fig 11.3: Cartoon by James Gillivray emphasising the agony experienced by a gout sufferer. (Courtesy The Wellcome Library, London.)

- King Henry VIII (1491–1547) – probably the most famous sufferer,
- Sir Isaac Newton (1643–1727) – a key player in the scientific revolution,

- Samuel Johnson (1709–84) who wrote that 'it has made me [as] helpless as an infant',
- Benjamin Franklin (1706–90) – a founding-father of the USA, of whom it was apparently written: 'You have indulged these legs of yours in indolence',
- Charles Dickens (1812–70) the celebrated author, who referred to the malady in *Pickwick Papers* (*see* Prologue), and much later
- Laurence (Baron) Olivier (1907–89),the English actor, who was apparently 'shaken' with gout.[25]

Significant additions, as well as numerous others, could include William Harvey (1578–1657) – discoverer of the systemic blood circulation – and Judge Jeffreys (1645–89), the 'hanging judge'.

Apart from an *hereditary* element, pre-disposition to gout has been largely unexplained; although 'rich man's gout' has been associated *historically* with an excessive intake of *port wine*, which of course contains a great deal of '*refined-sugar*'. One has only to read *'The Diary of a Country Parson'* (1758–1802) to appreciate the colossal consumption of port in the *eighteenth* century![26] It is of interest to recall that during *fructose*, but *not* glucose, metabolism, serum uric acid is significantly raised (*see* Chapter 8). Should the evolutionary/historical hypothesis outlined in Chapter 4 prove to be correct, it is clear that *fructose* will itself be shown responsible. Alcohol has also been linked to *gout* – the 'disease of kings' – accompanied by hyperuricemia and subsequent uric acid deposition in affected joints – but there is also evidence that obesity itself is in some way related to the disease, as is: red meat and 'junk food'.[27]

Obesity – produced by '*refined-sugar*' in numerous foodstuffs, sugary drinks included, is thus an *independent* risk-factor in causation of gout, and is associated with an earlier age of onset; likelihood of gout is virtually doubled in the obese, compared with those of normal weight.[28] The link is probably associated with increased *insulin-resistance*, associated with hyperuricemia in the obese, although the elevation of blood uric acid might occasionally result from renal failure.

Complications of obesity, including gout, also figured in another article: oversized women were welcomed by various bodies, including the British government which, it continued, was at that time still dithering over imposition of a *sugar tax* (*see* Chapter 16); clothes which would only fit *extremely* fat women who have, it claimed, a *reduced* average life-expectancy for the first time since the *nineteenth* century. This, according to the writer, arises from '... modern *liberal* insistence of celebrating every human failure as if it were a triumph'! But why should *gout* be more unacceptable than obesity itself, the article asked. While an increase in frequency of gout is *frightening*, we apparently still accept without question an increase in the incidence of obesity![29]

An extremely surprising and paradoxical finding is that an investigation in Sweden – published in *Rheumatology* – demonstrated a *lower* risk of arthritis in obese men; although the cause is unclear, that might relate to the *type* of masculine fat, or that this was *not* caused by sugar![30]

Dementia

Dementia, in a population of older people – the mean age of which is rapidly increasing – has recently received widespread attention, and there have in consequence been numerous articles on the subject in the British media. An association with obesity has recently become a matter of intense interest. An article in the *Postgraduate Medical Journal* for 2014 carried out by epidemiologists at the *University of Oxford,* which involved 'almost half a million hospital admissions in England since 1999', indicated that obesity in middle-aged individuals poses a *dementia* risk of about 50%, and that as younger cases of obesity become more common, the greater will that risk become! In fact, this incidence seemed to be age-related.[31] Conclusion(s) from that report were however challenged in a later study published in *Lancet Diabetes and Endocrinology* involving two million individuals; results from that report are directly contradictory to the previous finding.[32] Clearly, more studies on this crucially important matter are required, but the investigation should not be confused with memory loss and risk of dementia associated with *diabetes mellitus* (*see* above).[33]

A recent article, published in the journal *Neurobiology of Ageing* suggested that obesity can in fact age the brain by up to a decade. Clearly, further research should also be devoted to this subject.[34]

Malignancy

In 2014, a *Times* headline commenting on a report published in *Lancet Oncology* declared that in Britain: '**Being too fat causes cancer in 20,000 people every year**' (*see* fig 11.4).[35] Another claimed: 'Being overweight raises [the] cancer risk by up to 60%'. The latter study, carried out at the *London School of Hygiene and Tropical Medicine*, was based on 'health records of over five million adults in the UK over an average of 7½ years' in which it was demonstrated that body-weight was a risk factor for *ten* common cancers'. While the majority of malignancies were attributed simply to 'bad luck' (two thirds being caused by random mutations), the remainder were, it claimed, probably a result of lifetyle choices;[37] *sugar* in red meat, such as steaks and sausages, the report concluded, is for example probably responsible for some tumours, but others have a more indirect cause.[38] A study at the *University of California, San Diego* also suggested that it is the sugar in red meat which is responsible for an increased risk of cancer.

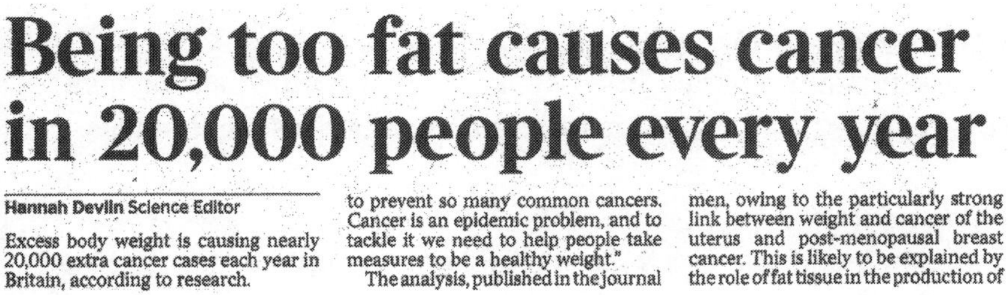

Being too fat causes cancer in 20,000 people every year

Hannah Devlin Science Editor

Excess body weight is causing nearly 20,000 extra cancer cases each year in Britain, according to research.

to prevent so many common cancers. Cancer is an epidemic problem, and to tackle it we need to help people take measures to be a healthy weight."

The analysis, published in the journal

men, owing to the particularly strong link between weight and cancer of the uterus and post-menopausal breast cancer. This is likely to be explained by the role of fat tissue in the production of

Fig 11.4: Headline in an article in the London *Times* newspaper (2014; November 26: 15) recording an association between obesity and malignancy.

One in every five (which could well be an underestimate) of 'cancer' deaths is apparently associated, concluded an *American Society of Clinical Oncology* meeting at Chicago, with obesity, and this is 'on track' to overtake smoking as the principal cause of malignant disease – breast and prostatic carcinoma being foremost, although colonic and gynaecological cancers were also mentioned. It was suggested that 'there [will] probably [be] a lag of *twenty years* between the obesity epidemic and [a rise in] cancer rate in the western world'.[39] Another conclusion was that in 'cancer patients', the chances of dying [were reduced by exercise] by up to 50 per cent'. A 'strong link' had also been recorded between being overweight or *obese* and presenting with 'advanced' prostate cancer; this association was based on multiple reviews of 104 studies involving 9.8 million men.[40]

On a more optimistic note, there is increasing evidence that daily aspirin (75mg) cancels the 'cancer-risk' of *obesity*; this conclusion was made as a result of a study involving almost 1000 individuals with Lynch syndrome†††* published in the *Journal of Clinical Oncology*.[41]

ANIMAL STUDY
An animal study is largely confirmatory. In mice, an aggressive form of breast malignancy was prevented by reducing calorie intake by 30%. This result reported in *Breast Cancer Research and Treatment*, will be followed by trials in women.[42]

Another association
An investigation reported in 2016 and carried out in Canada suggested that multiple sclerosis (MS) is more common in obese individuals.[43]

Conclusion(s)
So common and numerous are the systemic complications of obesity – especially *type-2-diabetes mellitus* – that, as well as inconvenience to the afflicted, the cost to the British NHS is huge – so great in fact that unless the prevalence of obesity is urgently reduced, it will become virtually impossible to maintain a Health Service in Britain!

††† Lynch syndrome is an inherited genetic disorder in which affected individuals have a higher than normal chance of developing: colorectal, breast or prostate cancer.

References and notes

1 J Yudkin. *Pure, white and deadly: how sugar is killing us and what we can do to stop it.* London: Penguin Books 1986: 126–141; (*See also*: Anonymous. Millions face obesity diseases, scientists fear. *Times, Lond* 2016; June 20: 18; N Mowbray. Wrinkles, red eyes, acne: the rise of 'sugar face'. *Times 2, Lond* 2016; May 10: 6–7; Anonymous. Obesity damages liver. *Times, Lond* 2016; June 17: 24; H Rumbelow. The Scandi Diet: delicious food and a flat stomach in twelve weeks. *Times 2, Lond* 2017; January 2: 2–3: 4–5.)

2 C Smyth. One in three now at risk as diabetes levels soar. *Times, Lond* 2014; 10 June: 1–2. K Gibbons. Four million Britons have diabetes. *Ibid* 2016; September 13: 22; C Smyth. Diabetes crisis costs the NHS £10 bn a year. *Ibid* 2016; January 5: 12; (*See also*: C Smyth. Diabetes death rate among young British men doubles in 15 years. *Ibid* 2015; 28 April: 6; K Lay. Diabetes patients take up a sixth of hospital beds. *Ibid* 2015 August 25: 2; K Lay. One in ten at high risk of diabetes. *Ibid* 2015; August 26: 21; S Nancollas. Modern 'leprosy'. *Ibid* 2015; September 3: 28; C Smyth. GPs spending £1 bn a year on insulin treatments. *Ibid* 2017; August 2: 12.)

3 M Stubbs. Diabetes epidemic. *Ibid* 2014; 12 June: 33; Anonymous. Two sugary drinks a day double risk of diabetes. *Ibid* 2016; October 21: 9; Anonymous. Child diabetes figures reveal obesity time bomb. *Ibid* 2017; August 12: 4.

4 K Gibbons. Half a billion people suffer in 'silent explosion' of diabetes. *Ibid* 2016; April 7: 4; Anonymous. Silent killer: an epidemic of diabetes requires co-ordinated action. *Ibid* 2016; April 7: 27; C Smyth. Diabetes hits obese young. *Ibid* 2016; June 15: 28.

5 K Lay, C Smyth. Depression and diabetes increase risk of dementia. *Ibid* 2015: February 21: 11.

6 A Satija, D Spiegelman, E Giovannucci, F B Hu. Type 2 diabetes and risk of cancer: strong evidence points to an association between diabetes and several major cancers. *Br med J* 2015; 350 (January 10): 8.

7 O Moody. Antibiotics linked to increased risk of developing diabetes. *Times, Lond* 2015: August 28: 17. (*See also*: Anonymous. Type 2 diabetes linked to higher antibiotic use. *Br med J* 2015; 351 [September 5]: 5.)

8   M Porter. If you're carrying too much weight, then diabetes is a serious risk. *Times 2, Lond* 2014; July 8:6.

9   O Moody. Fat diabetics 'outlive thinner ones'. *Times, Lond* 2015; May 5: 19.

10 K Gibbons. It's not what you eat, it's when you eat that really matters. *Ibid* 2016; June 22: 6.

11 C Smyth. Mother's milk helps reduce diabetes risk. *Ibid* 2015: December 4: 32; K Gibbons. Low-carb diet helps to control diabetes. *Ibid* 2016; May 31: 1, 6; C Askew. Diabetes and sugar. *Ibid* 2016; March 19: 22.

12 S Elks. Food plans curb threat of diabetes. *Ibid* 2015; June 11: 19;

13 C Smyth. Daily yoghurt may cut risk of diabetes. *Ibid* 2014; November 25: 24; O Moody. Daily glass of red wine can help diabetics. *Ibid* 2015; October 13: 20; Anonymous. Cholesterol reduces risk of diabetes. *Ibid* 2015: March 11: 17; M Mosley. Eight weeks, 800 calories a day: the diet that could save your life. *Times 2, Lond* 2016; June 2: 4–5.

14 A Milton. Control of diabetes. *Times, Lond* 2015; August 25: 28; O Moody. Failure to manage diabetes 'could bankrupt NHS'. *Ibid* 2015; August 17: 11. (*See also*: J Webb. Rugby star shows us how to tackle diabetes. *Ibid* 2015; August 21: 24.)

15 H McGuire, D Longson, A Adler, A Farmer, I Lewin. Management of type 2 diabetes in adults: summary of updated NICE guidance. *Br med J* 2016; 353: 73–4; C Askew. Action on diabetics. *Times, Lond* 2016; September 21: 30; S Hazel. Mind game tricks diabetics into controlling blood sugar. *Ibid;* 2016: July 16: 20; K Lay. Losing weight can reverse diabetes without drugs. *Ibid* 2017; December 6: 22. (*See also*: O Moody. Berries and chocolate could stave off diabetes. *Ibid* 2017; November 10: 9.)

16 T Whipple. Diabetes is 'cured' after gastric band operations. *Ibid* 2015; December 2: 4; K Gibbons. 'Instant' cure weight-loss surgery denied to diabetics. *Ibid* 2016; May 25: 6. (*See also*: T Whipple. Fasting diet could prove the cure for type 2 diabetes. *Ibid* 2017; February 24: 6; O Moody. Diabetes boot camp gets results. *Ibid* 2017; March 16: 21; Anonymous. Scientists halt diabetes with insulin cells. *Ibid* 2016; January 26: 23.)

17 K Dowling. Catastrophe as diabetes hits overfed felines. *Sunday Times, Lond* 2014: June 15: 15.

18 K Mansey, J Ungoed-Thomas. Children's sugar diet linked to heart disease. *Ibid* 2014; June 29: 10; M McCarthy. Higher sugar intake is linked to raised risk of cardio vascular mortality. *Br med J* 2014; February 8: 5; Anonymous. Reducing sugary drinks is linked to raised HDL levels. *Times, Lond* 2015; 351: 5; O Moody. Two sugary drinks a day can raise the risk of heart disease. *Ibid* 2015; November 3: 17. (See also: T Whipple. Sugar industry 'halted research after heart link'. *Ibid* 2017; November 22: 17.)

19 J Ungoed-Thomas. Sugar blamed for pumping up blood pressure. *Sunday Times, Lond* 2014; September 14: 8; C Smyth. Sensible diet cuts heart attack risk within weeks. *Times, Lond* 2015; March 19: 27; C Smyth. GPs told to give out blood pressure pills to cut heart attacks. *Ibid* 2015; December 24: 12.

20 M Porter. So, is high blood pressure caused by too much salt in your diet … or sugar? *Times 2, Lond* 2014; September 16: 6.

21 K Lay. High blood pressure is linked to greater risk of developing diabetes. *Times, Lond* 2015: September 29: 17.

22 C Smyth. Poor diet and lazy lives send stroke rate soaring among middle-aged men. *Ibid* 2015; May 12: 4.

23 C Smyth. Start walking and lose weight to prevent an epidemic of arthritis. *Ibid* 2014: September 6: 4.

24 I Torjesen. Rates of gout in the UK have increased but GP care has not improved. *Br med J* 2014; 348; 18 January: 2–3; R Hughes. Gout. *Times, Lond* 2014; January 20: 29; S Tharston. Gout. *Ibid* 2014; January 20: 29; S Stirling-Aird. Gout. *Ibid* 2014; January 27: 29. (*See also*: Anonymous. Gout dashed by diet. *Ibid* 2016: August 15: 4.)

25 C Smyth. Gout is no laughing matter for the portly: obesity blamed for huge rise as 'disease of kings' now afflicts more than a million. *Ibid* 2014; January 16: 19. (*See also*: C Smyth. Cheap meat blamed for return of gout. *Ibid* 2015; October 28: 17.)

26 J Woodforde. *The Diary of a Country Parson.* London: The Folio Society 1992: 445.

27 Op cit. *See* note 25 above.

28 C Smyth. Obesity and drinking fuel dramatic increase in gout. *Times,*

Lond 2014; July 24: 4.

29 G Coren. Why we shouldn't big up fat fashion. *Ibid* 2014; January 18: 22.

30 K Wright. Arthritis in knees is a preventable disease, scientists discover. *Ibid* 2017; August 15: 1, 2; K Lay. Obesity can reduce risk of developing arthritis in men. *Ibid* 2015; September 9: 19.

31 C Smyth. Slim to reduce the risk of dementia, middle-aged told. *Ibid* 2014; August 21: 14; K Lay. Having too much sugar could cause Alzheimer's. *Ibid* 2017; February 24: 15.

32 C Smyth. Eating too much sugar could make men depressed. *Ibid* 2017; July 28: 4; C Smyth. Fat middle-aged people have lower risk of dementia. *Ibid* 2015: April 10: 25.

33 Anonymous. Diabetes hits memory. *Ibid* 2015; July 9: 18; K Lay, C Smyth. Depression and diabetes increase risk of dementia. *Ibid* 2015; February 21: 11.

34 O Moody. Being overweight ages the brain by a decade. *Ibid* 2016; August 5: 16.

35 H Devlin. Being too fat causes cancer in 20,000 people every year. *Ibid* 2014: November 26: 15; K Lay. Mediterranean diet 'cuts cancer risk by 40%". *Ibid* 2017; March 6: 4; K Lay. Obesity linked to higher risk of 11 cancers. *Ibid* 2017; March 1: 20; Anonymous. Weight gain can triple cancer risk. *Ibid* 2017; February 15: 18; C Smyth. Lose stone and a half to reduce cancer risk. *Ibid* 2017; December 9: 4; (*see also* K Lay. Waist size could predict risk of developing cancer. *Ibid* 2017; May 24: 16; K Lay. Obesity fuels increase in kidney cancer. *Ibid* 2017; April 24: 18.)

36 V Forster. Being overweight raises cancer risk by up to 60%. *Ibid* 2014; August 14: 8; K Gibbons. Lose weight and get active to beat cancer, experts say. *Ibid* 2016; June 6: 4; Anonymous. Fruit cuts teenagers' cancer risk. *Ibid* 2016; February 1: 7.

37 H Devlin. Most cancer cases are just bad luck. *Ibid* 2015: January 2: 1, 5.

38 H Devlin. Sugar in red meat is blamed for increasing risk of cancer. *Ibid* 2014; December 30: 17; K Lay. Families give up meat over health fears. *Ibid* 2016; February 18: 1,5; T Whipple. Let your liver rest for two days every week, drinkers are told. *Ibid* 2016; January 2:

4; T Whipple. Better diet and more exercise can cut cancer deaths by 60%. *Ibid* 2016; June 23: 16.

39 C Smyth. Obesity fuels cancer deaths: fat to overtake smoking as leading cause of disease. *Ibid* 2015: May 30: 1,2.

40 Anonymous. Obesity is linked to advanced prostate cancer. *Ibid* 2014; November 19: 28; K Gibbons. Inches lost from waist cut prostate cancer risk. *Ibid* 2016; June 2: 1,2.

41 K Lay. Aspirin could cancel out cancer risk of being obese. *Ibid;* 2015; August 18: 8.

42 Anonymous. Sugary diet poses risk of breast cancer. *Ibid* 2016; January 2: 13; N Woolcock. Weight loss helps to beat breast cancer. *Ibid* 2014; May 26: 4.

43 Anonymous. MS linked to obesity. *Ibid* 2016; June 29: 14.

PART III:

Management of obesity

CHAPTER 12:

Management: the respective rôles of diet and exercise
(*see also*: Chapters 1–4)

Every strategy to tackle obesity must ultimately involve an impact on *energy balance.* This can best be brought about by:

- *Diet*: reduction of *calorie* intake – usually by restricting consumption of '*refined-sugar*', and/or
- *Exercise*: greater output of *calories*; how this is achieved is largely immaterial.

Both will be addressed in this and the following chapters. But before enlarging on this topic, it is of value to identify groups at risk:

Who is subject to obesity?
Researchers at the *University of Sheffield* have identified six distinct categories of being overweight:

- Young girls attempting to keep 'weight in check',
- Young men with high levels of alcohol consumption, and above average levels of physical activity,
- Unhappy and anxious middle-aged individuals – mostly female – who undertake moderate physical activity,
- Contented elderly individuals suffering from a severe physical debility – *eg,* osteoarthritis, hypertension and/or diabetes,
- Affluent elderly individuals – with above average alcohol intake, frequently accompanied by hypertension, and
- Those suffering from poor general health, lacking a healthy lifestyle and most not falling into the other groups.

It was envisaged that each group requires a different *preventive* solution.[1]

Dietary restriction

In *biblical* times, occasional (naturally occurring) honey was virtually the sole sweetener in the diet of *Homo sapiens* (*see* Chapter 5). When *refined-sugar* (sucrose) became available (*see* Chapter 6) it was initially a luxury and also very expensive. Only much later did its price plummet and it became no longer a luxury and confined in the rich and upper strata of society. During the last few decades, '*refined-sugar*' has become a *cheap* dietary component consumed by rich and poor alike. Some families, according to the President of the *Faculty of Public Health*, are now simply *not* able to afford a decent diet, and in consequence cheap processed food (including excessive '*refined-sugar*') is replacing a nutritious one – which of course includes fruit and vegetables. In fact *sugary* foods are now readily affordable by poorer sections of society – despite the fact that these same individuals are usually able to run at least one or more cars often as a '*prestige gimmick*'! According to the *Lancet*, amongst other sources, children especially are thus being fed on cheap food (containing an excess of '*refined-sugar*') which although filling, is far from nutritious.[2]

How much 'refined-sugar' *should both children and adults ingest?*
This was a question posed by the World Health Organisation (WHO) and London's *Sunday Times* newspaper in early 2014. It summarised anticipated differences of opinion between *Action on Sugar* (an organisation opposed to excessive dietary '*refined-sugar*') and the *World Sugar Research Organisation* (representing the *food industry*). A major concern however was '… whether policy makers [were] receiving *independent* advice on sugar intake?'

The consensus of opinion of a group of almost 2,000 from the latter group questioned by *YouGov* was that average consumption of '*refined-sugar*' was 'about right', it imposing only a 'modest risk' to health, and therefore a sugar *tax* should be opposed.[3]

Whereas *five* portions of fruit and vegetables daily in a healthy diet is now widely recommended to maximise longevity and in cardiac disease prevention, a study that *more* than this (*see* Chapter 7) will impart even more profound advantageous results had given negative results. This resulted from a review of 16 'high quality' investigations conducted by the *Harvard School of Public Health*, involving 833,000 people of more than 26 years. Whether or not this result applies to issues other than *obesity* remains unclear. As well as cardiac protection, a study at King's College London demonstrated that a healthy diet, *ie,* increased fruit and vegetables, and possibly reduction in fat, less 'fizzy drinks', as well as limitation of sweets and cakes is also compatible with weight-reduction. Following twelve weeks on this diet, average weight reduction was 1.3 kg, together with lessening of waistline by 0.7 cm, compared with weight gain of 0.6 and waist gain of 1.1 cm in a *control* group eating a 'typical British diet'. The beneficial effect of a low *'refined-sugar'* diet in prevention of cardiovascular mortality is also strongly suggested by research carried out by a *National Health and Nutrition Survey* and published in the journal *JAMA Internal Medicine.*[5]

A new product is the 'smart drink', consumption of which is a fast-growing nutritional trend; it is marketed to 'improve' 'brain-power'! Although described as a neuro-enhancing drink, whether this epithet can in fact be justified is open to question. One should certainly ask whether it is effective or not. Also, is this yet another 'health' product which has *obesity* as a side-effect?[6]

Women with eating disorders are apparently consuming increased volumes of wine and spirits (the calorie content of which is clearly displayed), in lieu of food; this study concluded that it is considered easier to consume a recommended number of calories by consuming alcoholic drinks instead of eating![7]

Both excessive wine and also 'junk food' input have been blamed for the striking increase in incidence of *gout* (*see* Chapter 11), and metabolism of *fructose* (*see* Chapter 8) might well be the answer. Although *genetic* factors are involved, no less than 86,866 hospital admissions in 2013–14 were related to *gout*; a figure compared with 48,717 in the previous five years, according to the *Health and Social Care Information Centre. Gout* is no longer therefore a disease of the rich and aristocratic as it was during the reign of King Henry VIII (1491–1547) for example, but is now a frequent cause of hospital admission especially in poorer sections of the British population.[8]

Individuals on any diet, incidentally tend to consume an *increase* in calories either *before* or in anticipation of a bout of exercise (*see* below); that increase is often higher than the permitted calorie intake. Researches from Boston and Taiwan – results of which were published in the *Journal of Health Psychology* – claimed that this *psychological* justification accounts for an *increase* in weight in some dieters who also take exercise.[9]

DOES A HIGH-FAT DIET CONTRIBUTE TO OBESITY?

Details of research on the effect of dietary fat have been provided in a book by Nina Teicholz *The Big Fat Surprise*[‡‡‡*] (*see* Chapter 4). The conclusion is consistent with numerous other observations and experience of dieters.[10] An article in *Open Heart* also cast serious doubt on official advice given in 1983 – designed to *reduce* dietary saturated *fat*. Advice was that only 30% of energy intake (including 10% of the saturated variety), should be in the form of *fat*, a conclusion from a careful study of trials then available which apparently contained 'serious gaps'. Although advice was aimed largely at reduction of arterial disease and blood cholesterol concentrations, it was also presumably applicable to obesity.[11] In an article by Ridley in 2014, it was also pointed out that this reduction was synonymous with *increased* '*refined-sugar*' – and its numerous complications.[12]

LABELLING OF FOOD

Advertised '*refined-sugar*' concentrations of foods available in supermarkets do *not* necessarily disclose the real amount, and numerous concentrations are in fact much higher than WHO guidelines, *ie,* to limit sugar content to 5% of energy intake. It is thus impossible for '… consumers to be able to make an informed choice'. But, 'From December 2016 it has [definitely] been *mandatory* for food companies to provide nutritional labelling [*see* below] on their products'; the relevant article recorded that *public health* can thus assist.[13]

To give an idea of the extent of the emotive 'lobby' working behind food *labelling*, an example from Paris is of note. Levels of obesity are presently lower in France than Britain, and the country's health minister has decreed that *all* items of food on sale *must* contain an indication – usually a colour code – of sugar content, in addition to that of salt, fat and total calories. However, that has provoked several claims that the move 'would be a disaster for [the] national cuisine', one objection being that 'Honey [will] get a red label, although [in the eyes of most it] is *good* for … health'.[14] The Chief Executive of the British supermarket *Morrisons* has suggested a novel strategy for increasing fruit consumption. All fruit on sale will, in future, be carefully packed and sold to the customer in *excellent* condition

---

‡‡‡ Arguably one of the most important books on nutrition.

as advertised, this reaction being in reply to the question: 'Who wants to give their kids bruised bananas to take to school?' As a result, it is hoped that *all* parents will give children *fresh* fruit instead of sugar-laden food.[15]

Reduction of 'fizzy drinks' (see also Chapter 3)

In June 2014, the front page of the London *Times* newspaper contained an article written by its health correspondent – '*Fizzy drinks are target in new war on sugar*'. This is a matter in which *public health* measures could assist. Under tough health guidelines, he wrote, 'Fizzy drinks would be effectively banished from the nation's diets'. This article was especially targeted towards children's drinks (*see* Table 12.1), and based on a review made by the *Scientific Advisory Committee on Nutrition*. '*Fizzy drinks*' should be replaced by water and fresh fruit. *Public Health England*, the article continued, was also considering the following measures:

Table 12.1: Weight (per 100 ml) of '*refined-sugar*' contained in 'fizzy' drinks

Colas

Coca Cola	10.6
Fentimans Curiosity Cola	11.3
Lidl Freeway Cola	10.9
Sainsbury's Classic	10.8
Essential Waitrose	10.7

Sparkling elderflower drinks

Schloer White Grape and Elderflower	10.7
Pure Pret Grape and Elderflower	10.6

Ginger beers

Old Jamaica	15.7
Barr's Originals	14.1
Waitrose	13.9
Marks & Spencer Fiery	13.8
Fentimans	9.4

- a sugar tax (*see* Chapter 16), initially opposed by government,
- limits on portion sizes of all sugary foods,
- restrictions on advertising, and
- banning discounted chocolates.[16]

Controls on 'fizzy drinks' advertising, together with health warnings on food products with a high '*refined-sugar*' content are other recommendations. However, the same article reported that although government was determined to reduce '*refined-sugar*' consumption, it 'had *no* plans at that time to introduce a sugar tax' (*see* Chapter 16). Furthermore, 'the sugar industry had warned that 'proposals to cut sugar intake to … 5% of calories could make people even fatter, for the simple reason that cutting sugar *intake* could lead to a higher intake of [both] fatty and higher calorie foods'.[17] Another article in the London *Times* newspaper focused on '*refined-sugar*' concentration of '… ginger beer and sparkling elderflower drinks …' which might be consumed at a picnic.[18] One other recommendation by *Public Health England* was that 'Parents should [provide] a jug of water on the table at mealtimes rather than serve children with juice and 'fizzy drinks' …'. Also, was the realisation that 'manufacturers of energy drinks … promoted the fallacy that *sugary drinks* were healthy, placing pressure to buy (*via* peer persuasion) trendy *sports drinks'*.[19]

Efficacy of Public Health campaigns
Whereas in 1978 only 7% of the English population was *obese*, by 2014 this figure amounted to more than 25%, a further third being merely deemed overweight. These figures affected children in particular, and one solution would be to get infants and children walking as soon as possible – in fact to give up the buggy! Lack of physical activity (*see* below) coupled with an unhealthy diet is likely to exert a disastrous effect on future generations (*see* below). The author quoted a recent article in *The New England Journal of Medicine* indicating that 'half [50%] of obese children are destined to become obese adults …'. This is similar to experience with the '*new tobacco*'; it will be recalled that it required about thirty years from the first reports of adverse effects, to widespread acceptance of an association between smoking and bronchial carcinoma.[20]

Past failures of preventive medicine

There has, during the last few decades been a failure of *preventive medicine* to find an adequate solution to the problem of escalating sugar consumption. It had become obvious, certainly since the 1960s, when Yudkin launched his 'crusade' against *'refined-sugar'*, that this dietary product was exerting a deleterious effect on the health of *H sapiens*, especially during the first few years of life. What then have previous *Chief Medical Officers* (CMO)s – who are after all ultimately guardians of the nation's health, and answerable to the UK government – achieved? Another unassociated disaster, completely unrelated to diet, and *not* tackled over many decades is that of antibiotic-resistance[21], which only the present CMO has attempted to tackle. Previous attention has been placed *only* on a diminution of tobacco consumption. CMOs should appreciate that there are numerous *other* health problems, accepting that *'refined-sugar'* is perhaps the most important of these!

The present situation regarding influence of *'refined-sugar'* on health has also been seriously hampered by the UK's failure to raise *human nutrition* to the status of an independent *specialty* – an *academic* discipline. To my personal knowledge, this issue has been aired on numerous occasions and repeatedly rejected by powerful individuals – some within the medical profession; it has been 'shelved off' to other specialist bodies to implement. Of all specialties, this discipline, important to every member of *H sapiens* throughout the world, is surely worthy of independent *academic* status.

Government is primarily interested in the economy, business, employment, and more importantly value of shares; *health* has either been of limited or of *no* concern until for example, the escalating cost of *type-2-diabetes* which is threatening to destroy the *National Health Service* (NHS). A high profile debate in May 2014 on whether *Pfizer* would subsume the British pharmaceutical company *AstraZeneca* is a further example. This debate surrounded business aspects – including USA taxes; the fact that *AstraZeneca*'s excellent *Research and Development* (R&D) programme was in serious jeopardy received only scant attention. Profit and shareholders were both deemed of paramount importance; the fact that development of *new* therapeutic compounds could be in danger barely entered the discussion![22]

The General Practitioner's rôle in halting the obesity epidemic
Another potential strategy is to arrange for general practitioners to offer weight-management courses (*eg, Weight Watchers* or *Slimming World*) to *all* overweight/obese patients (*see* Chapter 2); this recommendation was also made in guidance from the *National Institute for Health and Care Excellence* (NICE).[23] 'Competitive dieting' is another approach to weight-reduction, friends being supportive of others' efforts to reduce weight; such a 'mutual support' strategy, although initially valuable, has however been shown to diminish with time, according to an American study published in the *Journal of Consumer Research*.[24]

A timely editorial in the *Times* newspaper focusing on the *obesity epidemic*, concluded that 'people in wealthy countries now suffer from diseases resulting from lifestyle changes rather than on poverty [unlike the situation in the *nineteenth* century]'.[25] That this is *not* entirely the government's responsibility was emphasised by a British Health Minister: 'Individuals... should take responsibility for [personal] wellbeing by adjusting their lifestyle(s).'[26] The fact that being overweight is now frequently considered 'normal' (*see* Preface) has been emphasised by Britain's CMO; she has again appealed for both 'clearer labelling' of food products (*see* above), and also that food and drink manufactures should 'use [significantly] less *added* sugar'.[27]

An article quoting a Professor of *Public Health & Policy* at the *University of Liverpool*, claimed that halving the '[number] of sweetened drinks consumed by British children could [reduce] intake by up to 100 calories a day'; he has suggested 'compulsory labelling' (*see* above and Chapter 3) of *all* sugary drinks, especially those aimed at children.[28]

AN OBESITY TAX

It is estimated that 'dealing with long-term consequences of obesity presently costs the NHS around £5.1 billion [annually]'. A *tobacco* tax (*see* Chapter 16) went a long way to saving the NHS. In the same way, a tax on 'drivers of obesity' (*ie,* the *sugar industry*), if and when imposed, would to some extent solve the 'moral dilemma' associated with refusal of treatment for the obese.[29] This would also act as a catalyst for the *industry* to reduce '*refined-sugar*' in their products.'

Attempts to reduce weight by dietary means in the already obese
Rôle of dieting

While dietary restrictions should be similar to those for *prevention* of obesity, these have perhaps been less clearly defined in the media.

As was correctly pointed out from a dietician in a letter to the *Times* in 2014, the human diet contains numerous sugars, but that associated with obesity is almost certainly *fructose* (which constitutes *50% of sucrose*); the others, including milk sugar (lactose) are considered *not* to play a part![30] However, to illustrate another viewpoint, a Nutritionist and Nutrition Communications Manager at *'Sugar Nutrition, UK'* had written, a mere fortnight before:

> ... Expert committees, including the *WHO European Food Safety Authority* and *UK Department of Health* have reviewed scientific evidence over many years and *all* have concluded that the balance of available evidence does *not* [my italics] implicate [sucrose] in any of the so-called 'life-style diseases'.[31]

A return to biblical diets (which were detailed and could lead to weight reduction) was a recommendation in a *Times* leading article in late 2013 (*see* above).[32] Obviously, the first imperative in a dietary solution to the 'obesity epidemic' is to reduce dietary intake of obesogenic foodstuffs. First and foremost must be a reduction in *'refined-sugar'*, and a study at the *University of Reading* concluded that by incorporating 'sugar-free swaps' at meal times it was possible to reduce daily *'refined-sugar'* intake from 483 to 196 grammes.[33]

REDUCTION OF TOTAL CALORIFIC VALUE OF FOOD

A simple reduction in calorific value of ingested foodstuff seems good sense, but perhaps this solution is a little too naive and simplistic![34] The idea has received a pretty hostile response; restaurants should reduce the *size* of puddings, a government idea which applied not only to restaurants, but to cafés and pubs as well. This potential solution would in any case *not* automatically reduce amounts of *'refined-sucrose'* ingested.[35]

YOGHURT

The rôle of certain forms of yoghurt in reducing weight has recently come to the fore. In a study based on 8,500 normal (*ie, not* overweight) men and women; '*full-fat*' yoghurt seemed effective, but the *low-fat* version has had little impact – according to a group of Spanish researchers. The reason for the difference is not immediately clear, but could be because the *low-fat* variety contains more added '*refined-sugar*' to counteract diminished taste. There is also the possibility that colonic flora which have an effect on body-weight, might proliferate. It is known incidentally that certain genetic compositions favour weight-reducing colonic bacteria (*see* Chapter 4).[36]

FAT

Between the 1950s and 2014, the world's population was virtually 'compelled' to believe that fatty foods were contraindicated and that their frequent consumption was even counterproductive to longevity (*see* above and Chapter 4)! The fact that *fat* was to be avoided undoubtedly led to a significant *increase* in '*refined-sugar*' consumption.[37] As a result of this evidence, fat was largely replaced by '*refined-sugar*' as a *calorie* source. This *new* evidence was 'good news' to manufacturers who proceeded to concentrate on *benefits* of fatty diets. Nevertheless, there remained doubters, although in a minority, in the ranks! It was apparently admitted that it is 'quite difficult to interpret results of clinical trials in terms of dietary habits'.[38] Low-fat diets had not in any case led to weight-loss! The 'Atkins diet', which contains fat, is for example, associated with weight-loss!

Exercise – as a preventive strategy

Health (obesity included) of future generations is largely in the hands of the nation's parents. The Victorians cared far more about the *State of the Nation's Health* than is the case today. This era (1837–1901) saw cricket, soccer, rugby, cycling, tennis, and swimming increase in Britain substantially, both in participation and popularity, and thus thousands of sports facilities were established. Rather than overloading health-care with numerous cases of obesity – and its complications (*see* Chapter 4) – exercise was encouraged! It would therefore be more in line with historical achievements, if government were to invest far more in sports centres, swimming pools, and sports fields rather than the reverse which took place under Thatcher's government, when numerous playing fields were sold off – which like many other achievements when she was 'at the helm' – were disastrous.[39]

One English council education chief has suggested, amongst opposing views, that children should be compelled to *walk* to school, *ie,* parents should be made to park their cars 'at least half a mile [away] from schools'. This proposal, he claimed, was 'as much to help children as [their] parents to keep fit' and thus avoid obesity.[40] An Australian study of 204,000 men and women aged >45 years at the *James Cook University*, indicated that those who incorporated a 'workout' into their lifestyle had reduced mortality by 9–13%, and that the more strenuous the exercise the greater was the benefit. This applied also to individuals not necessarily obese, as well as those who already had obesity complications.[41] Short 'workouts' (*ie,* those lasting less than 20 minutes) incorporating considerable intensity *might* also be a key to weight-loss, *ie,* there is a 'rapid law of diminishing returns'.[42] Since 'intensity' training for long periods is known to be beneficial, it had previously been considered that advantageous effects of exercise were time-related. Another writer has suggested that daily walks with a dog not only prevent obesity in its owner, but also in the animal itself![43]

Can obesity be reversed?
Once obesity or overweightness has taken hold, it is of course extremely difficult to reverse:

- Elimination of excessive food and drink (including alcohol – especially beer), much containing '*refined-sugar*' (sucrose) (*see* above), and
- Increased exercise.

Addressing the second recommendation, one health correspondent has recommended, amongst other strategies, a 'brisk 30-minute walk [on] five days a week' which also acts beneficially on 'heart disease, hypertension, high cholesterol and diabetes …'. Anti-obesity effects of exercise have been stressed in another article with avoidance of *osteoarthritis* in mind; however, those with pre-existent cardiac disease are rightly advised to take a cautious approach. Questions however surround other strategies; although many solutions have been attempted few have a proven beneficial effect.[44]

Other possible strategies
Avoidance of breakfast – formerly felt to be a step on the path to *cure* of obesity – is no longer considered a satisfactory solution; in a study at *St George's Hospital, London*, three hundred overweight volunteers avoided breakfast during a 16-week period; the *conclusion* being that avoidance of breakfast had *no* discernible effect.[45]

There is also probably no truth in the recent idea that butter in coffee is a solution; this must remain suspect.[46]

The old adage that 'an apple a day keeps the doctor away' possibly has some relevance![47]

Conclusions
In a recent article in the London *Times 2* newspaper, Dr Michael Mosley attempted to destroy 10 *myths* concerning the difficult problem of obesity *prevention*. These are:

- Always eat breakfast,
- Set moderate weight goals,
- Crash diets are less successful than steady weight-loss,
- It is better to eat several small meals a day for weight-loss,
- Very-low-calorie eating slows down long-term metabolism,
- Diets based on fasting make you feel faint,
- Juicing diets are a good way to lose weight,
- Two litres of water a day will help weight-loss,
- Being overweight is healthy if <65 years old, and
- Any exercise will lead to weight-loss.

Each *myth* was given a detailed explanation, while most were accompanied by a relevant reference. The first was endorsed by several other investigators, the *conclusion* being that 'it's not ... *breakfast* calories but the total [that count] …'. Thus, yet another *myth* has hit the dust![48]

A major strategy set out by the Conservative Party in early 2013 (*ie, before* the 2014 General Election) (*see also* Chapter 2) was criticised by the *Lancet*. The issue which they opposed was that a long-term cure for obesity lay in *bariatric* surgery; to subject *all* sufferers of severe obesity to major surgery was considered both 'ethically and financially questionable' (*see* Chapter 15).

References and notes

1   K Lay. Six different types of obesity and as many ways treat it. *Times, Lond* 2015: April 18: 7.

2   C Smyth. Children going hungry in 'Oliver Twist Britain'. *Ibid* 2014; May 2: 25

3   J Ungoed-Thomas, K Mansey. Sugar advisers have their cake and eat it. *Sunday Times, Lond* 2014; January 19: 12.

4   C Smyth. More than five fruit and veg a day won't make you healthier. *Times, Lond* 2014; July 30: 19.

5   M McCarthy. Higher sugar intake is linked to raised risk of cardiovascular mortality. *Br med J* 2014; 348: 5; C Smyth. Sensible diet cuts heart attack risk within weeks. *Times, Lond* 2015; March 19: 27; K Lay. Putting on just a few pounds raises risk of dying early. *Ibid* 2017; July 19: 17; P Bee. This summer's cult beach diet: a seven-day crash programme that's been around since the Eighties is popular again. *Times 2, Lond* 2017; July 18: 7.

6   P Bee. Intelligence? They're bottling it; new 'smart drinks' are promising to improve our brain power. But can the claims be justified? *Times, Lond* 2014; July 8: 7.

7   R Bennett. 'Drinkorexics' lose weight by replacing food with alcohol. *Ibid* 2015; February 10: 21; C Smyth. Alcohol has no health benefits after all. *Ibid* 2015; February 11: 6.

8   C Smyth. Obesity and drinking fuel dramatic increase in gout. *Ibid* 2014; July 24: 4.

9   O Moody. Why dieters who exercise end up putting on weight. *Ibid* 2015; May 16: 17.

10 N Teicholz. *The Big Fat Surprise: why butter, meat and cheese belong to a healthy diet.* London: Scribe 2014; 369.

11 J Ungoed-Thomas, J Stoneman. Diet experts to put big fat lie in blender. *Sunday Times, Lond* 2016; June 12: 4.)

12 M Ridley. Experts have been feeding us a big fat myth: a new book shows that the low fat craze was based on flimsy evidence. Be wary of today's advice from the diet police. *Times, Lond* 2014; June 30: 25; M Ridley. Obesity dogma has done us a fat lot of good: some put on weight more easily than others and there is no point in being proscriptive until scientists are certain why. *Ibid* 2017; May 22: 25.

13 J Ungoed-Thomas. 'Healthy wholegrain' biscuits and cereals packed with sugar. *Sunday Times, Lond* 2017; February 19: 3.

14 A Sage. French delicacies to carry health warnings. *Times, Lond* 2014; June 20: 35.

15 D Walsh. Soft fruit is a weapon of choice in Morrisons' battle. *Ibid* 2014; June 27: 47.

16 C Smyth. Fizzy drinks are target in new war on sugar. *Ibid* 2014; June 27: 1,2.

17 K Mansey, J Ungoed-Thomas. Leaked report calls for tax onslaught on sugary drinks. *Sunday Times, Lond* 2014; June 15: 7.

18 O Moody. 'Middle-class' soft drinks contain most sugar. *Times, Lond* 2014; June 12: 13.

19 H Devlin. Serve water instead of fizzy drinks to cut obesity, parents told. *Ibid* 2014; June 26: 3.

20 J Russell. Beat obesity. Get your child out of that buggy. *Ibid*; June 12: 30.

21 G C Cook. Before the 'germ theory': a history of cause and management of infectious disease before 1900. Ely, Cambridgeshire: Melrose Books 2015: 202.

22 Anonymous. Pfizer's Dream: Pfizer has much to do to convince shareholders that its intent to take over AstraZeneca will ensure gains to UK investment and employment. *Times, Lond* 2014; May 7: 30.

23 O Moody. GPs get new weapon to fight obesity: the prescription diet. *Ibid* 2014; May 28: 14.

24 K Burgess. Dieter's camaraderie wears thin as pounds fall off. *Ibid* 2015; January 23: 13.

25 Anonymous. Public Health: making Britain healthier may be tough but people can still help themselves. *Ibid* 2013; August 28: 26.

26 G Bidsdale. Biblical diets. *Ibid* 2013; November 31: 27; Anonymous. The Good Cookbook: following the Daniel diet, how could the Bible inspire weight-loss. *Ibid* 2013: November 29: 32.

27 M Limb. Action is needed over "alarming" levels of obesity, says CMO. *Br med J* 2014; 348: 5; C Smyth. Now it's normal to be fat, warns Britain's health chief. *Times, Lond* 2014; March 28: 3.

28 Op cit. *See* note 13 above.

29 A Currie. Tax on obesity. *Times, Lond* 2016; December 1: 32.

30 E Roberts. Sugar rush. *Ibid* 2014; January 28: 29.

31 G Jones. Sugar. *Ibid* 2014 January 14: 27.

32 Anonymous. The Good Cookbook: following the Daniel diet, how else could the bible inspire weight loss? *Ibid* 2013; November 29: 32.

33 C Smyth. Dump the lumps with sugar swaps, urge health chiefs. *Ibid* 2015; January 5: 4.

34 D Aaronovitch. Forget the faddy diets and go back to basics: the debate over fat and carbs obscures the truth that consuming fewer calories than we burn is the only way to slim. *Ibid* 2015; February 23: 25.

35 C Smyth. Restaurant ordered to reduce size of puddings: Cut calories or be named and shamed, Hunt says. *Ibid* 2016; September 30: 1, 2; M Armstrong. Pudding purdah. *Ibid* 2016; October 1: 26; L Purves. Get your grimy spoon out of my pudding: Jeremy Hunt must stop prattling about supersized desserts and instead get to grips with the complex causes of obesity. *Ibid* 2016; October 3: 25; K Maher. Oi, Jeremy Hunt, keep your hands off my biscotti. *Times 2, Lond* 2016; October 3: 4.

36 K Lay. Lose weight with a designer yoghurt. *Times, Lond* 2014; November 7: 10; O Moody. Yoghurt cuts obesity but only if it's full-fat. *Ibid* 2014; May 31: 16.

37 D Housden. Saturated fat. *Ibid* 2015; February 12: 29; M Mosley. The full-fat diet – why it's not as unhealthy as you think. *Times 2, Lond* 2014; July 2: 2–3; Z Morris. Eat fat and get slim: the new diet plan to lose weight fast. *Ibid* 2015; January 3: 4–5; K Lay. Diet advice 'is not backed by evidence'. *Times, Lond* 2015; February 10: 6.

38 A Epstein. The truth about fats, the good, the bad and the fashion-able: dietary advice to cut out butter and full-cream milk is outdated and misguided, new research suggests. So which fats should we be eating? *Times 2, Lond* 2015: February 14: 4–5; K Lay. Fat can help to fight off heart disease. *Times, Lond* 2015; June 8: 12; K Lay. Low-fat diets don't boost weight loss chances. *Ibid* 2015; October 30: 18; Anonymous. Avoiding fat will not stop obesity, warn scientists. *Ibid* 2016; May 23: 18; J Duigan. Eat fat, lose weight: follow the trainers two-week diet plan: a new report says that eating fat can make you slim. *Times 2, Lond* 2016; May 28: 4–5; Anonymous. Food Fight:

public health officials should re-examine the conventional wisdom on fat. *Times, Lond* 2016; May 24: 29; D Lawson. Swap the sweet nothings for nature's healthiest option – fat, glorious fat. *Sunday Times, Lond* 2016; May 29: 24; K Gibbons. Bad cholesterol 'helps you live longer'. *Times, Lond* 2016; June 13: 8; Anonymous. Atkins diet heart risk. *Ibid* 2016; November 15: 4; O Moody. Professor who backed butter now says it's best avoided. *Ibid* 2016; July 20: 15.

39 K Chagger. Model Victorians. *Ibid* 2015; May 8: 34.

40 Anonymous. Call for curb on school run to tackle child obesity. *Ibid*; June 7: 9.

41 N Woolcock. Live longer with vigorous exercise, middle-aged told. *Ibid* 2015; April 7: 20.

42 A Radnor, R Gledhill. Bursts of exercise 'key to weight loss'. *Ibid* 2013: December 3: 10. (*See also*: K Lay. Half an hour of walking better than gym for losing weight. *Times, Lond* 2015; November 4: 1,9; P Bee. The myth of walking 10,000 steps: a brisk, daily 30-minute walk is better for us than the gym … Yet is that really enough? *Times 2, Lond* 2015; November 4: 2–3; W Pavia. One 60-minute run can add 7 hours to your life. *Times, Lond* 2017: April 14: 5.)

43 P Naughton. Fat dogs spur lazy owners into walkies. *Ibid* 2014; December 12: 25; O Moody. Want to live longer? Give a dog a home. *Ibid* 2017; November 18: 37.

44 C Smyth. Start walking and lose weight to prevent an epidemic of arthritis. *Ibid* 2014; September 6: 4; H Devlin. Exercise could kill you, heart patients warned. *Ibid* 2014; August 13: 4.

45 K Gibbons. Give breakfast a miss if you want to lose weight. *Ibid* 2016; March 25: 11; D Sanderson. Skip breakfast for a healthier brain. *Ibid;* April 1: 13.

46 R Blakely. For a shot at weight-loss, put butter in your coffee. *Ibid* 2014; December 16: 13

47 R Blakely. An apple a day: healthcare app will alert doctors to users' weighty issues. *Ibid* 2014; June 3: 45.

48 M Mosley. Crash diets, juicing and exercise: 10 myths about weight loss. *Times 2, Lond* 2014; June 14: 6–7;

Chapter 13:

Other 'non-invasive' strategies which possibly counteract obesity

Diet and increased exercise are the most obvious solutions for the individual (*see* Chapter 12). But there are others – especially in this era of technological advance – some of which are dealt with in this chapter.[1]

Reclassification of 'refined-sugar'
What would seem to be a sensible approach was outlined in a letter to the *Times* in early 2015. The writer suggested that food and drink 'full of sugars' should be reclassified by the government – *not* as foodstuffs, but as *confectionery*. In this case, higher VAT rating could be imposed, leading indirectly to a diet containing a high *'refined-sugar'* content becoming healthier!

The rôle of the General Practitioner
In early 2014, the *British Medical Journal* published an article suggesting that general practitioners should be more frank about dealing with weight problems. They should for example, implement much tougher *public health* messages: breakfast with an unsweetened cereal should be encouraged, together with other low-carbohydrate regimes, as should TV-free days. Increased exercise should also be addressed: a mere twenty minutes of brisk walking not only reduces weight but diminishes premature mortality by one-third. Coupled with such advice should be the fact that since the lungs constitute the primary excretory site in weight-limitation; physical exercise and deep breathing is a further solution to obesity!

Re-introduction of *public weigh-ins* has been recommended by some; and frequent assessment of results by their general practitioner might save the *National Health Service* (NHS) a great deal of money!

Further, attention to advice on exercise should be encouraged, and disposal of school sports fields (which has occurred in recent years) roundly condemned.

152

The undergraduate medical curriculum contains far too little emphasis on nutrition' and as a result, dietary advice to overweight patients is frequently lacking. Therefore, this should be given a far higher profile in medical training, having been 'down played' by several senior individuals in important consultative bodies.[2]

Other contributions
Psychological treatment and place of residence
A recent *Times* article stressed that obese individuals are sometimes treated by the NHS as 'second class citizens'; on occasion they have even been *refused* treatment! A suggestion that psychological therapy – comparable to that used to reduce *tobacco* consumption – perhaps obtainable on the NHS – will probably *not* solve the problem of excessive *'refined-sugar'* but might help.

Living near a busy road is also apparently a risk-factor.[3]

'Internet' diets
Weight-loss treatments, claimed to possess 'quick-fix' solutions – which can be purchased *via* the internet (most however, *not* designated 'authorised medicines') can cause dangerous side-effects. Also 'probiotic drinks' have been advocated and are said to have a market value worth £20 billion. However, evidence for their efficacy is lacking; this has been published in *Genome Medicine*. A 'food adulteration' scam, worth £1 billion annually, not *solely* connected with weight-reduction diets, has recently been uncovered by the *National Food Crime Unit*. Fraudulent food is frequently targeted towards adolescents attending music festivals etc.[4]

Office posture
It has been suggested that assuming a standing posture and introduction of 'standing desks' in offices might be beneficial as far as weight is concerned. Among those who have apparently preferred the 'standing desk' have included: Sir Winston Churchill (1874–1965) and the former US Defence Secretary Donald Rumsfeld (1932–present). However, further research has indicated that such a strategy is of only limited benefit.[5]

The 'coffee-shop habit', value of 'Green Tea, and supermarkets'
This part of Britain's lifestyle dates back to the coffee-shop culture of the *seventeenth* century. There has apparently been a 20% *increase* in coffee-shop branches over the last two decades. Often American in their origin(s), they can lead to *'piling on the pounds'*! On the other hand, taking 'green-tea' made from the shrub *Camellia sinensis* with every meal is said to assist 'weight-loss'; this apparently reduces calories absorbed from bread and potatoes, for example. The result was based on a controlled trial carried out in Poland and published in the journal *Scientific Report*. Interestingly; *full-fat* yoghurt reduces obesity by 20%, but the low-fat version has limited impact (*see* Chapter 12). This was concluded from a study in Spain involving 8,500 individuals who were *not* suffering from excessive weight or obesity, and it is likely that the difference was due to a higher 'sugar' content in low-fat yoghurt.[6]

In an attempt to reduce weight, especially in childhood, banning obesogenic foodstuffs at supermarket checkouts has been recommended by the *British Medical Association* (BMA). Although this strategy has been welcomed by several traders, it is too early to give a clear answer to its efficacy. By late 2014 *Tesco* had resolved to remove sweets and chocolates from all checkouts in its stores in Britain and in the Republic of Ireland. Another store (*Lidl*) went a step further in displaying fresh and dried fruit, oatcakes and juices close to their checkouts.[7]

Listen to yourself eating
An experimental strategy introduced by American psychologists is to listen to oneself chewing! This, the researchers concluded, was a sure way of losing weight.[8]

Plain packets for sweets
Mars (one of the world's largest confectionery companies) has apparently advised government ministers *against* plain packets for sweets and chocolates – in a way comparable to that of cigarettes. Such a strategy, it suggested, would simply promote 'an increase in counterfeit goods and consequently an *increase* in smuggling'.[9]

Awareness of an expanding waistband
Obesity, excessive drinking and lack of exercise currently costs the NHS approximately £11 billion annually; as a consequence, a £3 million advertising campaign has been launched. It is surmised that individuals who pay attention to health in their 40s and 50s are usually fit later on, but on the other hand it is never too late to apply weight-reduction. Awareness of an expanding waistband can now be measured with a 'smart-belt'.[10]

Changes to lifestyle
Avoidance of television, diets and coffee shops has been suggested in another move to counteract obesity. An amended lifestyle recommended by the *National Institute for Clinical Excellence* (NICE) includes the following:

- Avoid giving children sweets/chocolates as a 'reward',
- Limit TV viewing time,
- Substitute water for 'fizzy drinks' to quench thirst,
- Avoid fad diets and obsessive exercise,
- Breakfasting on a plain cereal with low-fat milk,
- Eat wholemeal bread, pasta and rice, and
- Consume meals as a family event.

Assistance using a 'high-tech' approach to weight-reduction in childhood, in an attempt to inculcate a healthy lifestyle – which can be used widely by schools – is another approach!

Assessment of calorie-intake
The brain automatically and subconsciously 'counts the calories'. Several 'new-tech' means of counting calories have recently come to the fore. A handheld scanner (the size of a pack of cards) can perform that function and *via* a molecular sensor assesses the calorie-count of both food and beverages. Also, based on the brain's ability to select suitable low-calorie foodstuffs, an experimental study published in *Psychological Science* correlated the brain's ability (*via* a brain scan) to a select list of items of diet – based on calorie content.

Another 'new' strategy is to track the daily 'number of bites of food'. A *bite monitor* has been perfected; this – in principle rather like a pedometer – is worn on the wrist like a watch and counts the number of bites into food. It is based on an estimate that one bite represents 17 calories for men and 11 for women; daily totals were 1,700 and 1,100 bites respectively. But such a simple device has apparently been criticised by several dieticians.

An American invention (the SmartPlate), claimed to accurately monitor numbers of calories ingested, consists of a plate with hidden television cameras on its side! Another portable device is a miniature DNA kit (the 'Bento lab') which reveals precise composition of a meal. Yet another is a 'smart plate' which counts total calories about to be consumed, this consisting of a plate containing three hidden digital cameras. Photographs are immediately relayed, and the images compared with known dietary constituents. Scanning a meal for an instant calorie-count is another 'high-tech' device.

A portable DNA kit which costs <£800 has recently been unveiled at a London laboratory. It monitors all dietary items and can reveal whether foodstuffs are genuine or not; it can also analyse samples of saliva and hair.[11]

Smaller plates to reduce calorie-intake

An argument has been put forward that reduction in the *size* of meals, plates and spoons reduces incidence of obesity. There is probably some truth in this and one estimate is that by elimination of the largest helpings, daily calorie intake could be reduced by an average of 16 per cent.[12]

Using a pill or injection to lessen obesity

According to a *Times* report, researchers at *Harvard University and Massachusetts Institute of Technology* have developed an injection to 'adjust a faulty gene that causes metabolism to burn ... excess fat'. That of course presupposes that the basic defect in obese individuals is genetic and *not* environmental! *Sibutramine* (Reductil) was in use until 2010, however in that year it was suspended following a review by the *European Medicine Agency* because cardiovascular risks were shown to outweigh benefits. A replacement would be welcome.[13]

Other measures to reduce incidence of obesity
Various other strategies to tackle the *obesity pandemic* have been suggested:

- Reduction of loneliness – especially in teenagers,
- Removal to a town, with a 'track record' of being associated with improved overall health, obesity included,
- Reduction in ambient temperature, *ie,* by 'turning down' central heating.
- A mirror in the dining room. A US study involving 185 undergraduates, showed that those offered a slice of chocolate cake, instead of a fruit salad, were far less likely to enjoy it if there was a mirror in the room!
- Sunbathing. A study in *mice* has demonstrated a slowing of weight gain following exposure to the sun. However, the mechanism, and its relevance to *Homo sapiens*, has *not*, to date, been demonstrated.

Other chapters in this book have outlined *preventive* and *curative* measures to counteract the current *obesity epidemic*, but several other *non-surgical* strategies have also been mentioned. However, many are guided by *calorie* input, often estimated by the individual concerned, although records are often erroneous – due either to inaccurate documentation or blatant dishonesty – and this chapter has drawn attention to various devices which *might* be of assistance.[14]

Diminution *of illegal 'refined-sugar' imports into Britain*
Recent evidence indicates that '*refined-sugar*' is entering Britain *illegally*. Kenyan troops serving in Somalia are reported to have been operating a 'sugar-smuggling racket' worth perhaps up to $400 million annually. Clearly this should be discontinued forthwith, and if necessary some form of punishment immediately instituted.[15]

References and notes

1   K Lay. Internet diet miracles can be deadly, warns watchdog. *Times, Lond* 2015; December 30: 4; T Whipple. Probiotic drinks dismissed as a waste of money for the healthy. *Ibid* 2016; May 10: 19; S-K Templeton. Doctors demand ban on unhealthy food at checkouts. *Sunday Times, Lond* 2015; July 12: 14; S Calman. Sweet nothings. *Times, Lond* 2015; August 5: 26.

2   K Gibbons. 'Inept' doctors failing to prescribe healthy eating for patients. *Ibid* 2016; June 10: 11; P Kidd. My cure for the obesity epidemic – public weigh-ins. *Times2, Lond* 2014; May 29: 2; C Smyth. GPs urged to weigh all patients in crackdown on obesity. *Times, Lond* 2016; October 15: 1,6; G Iacobucci. Incentivise GPs to tackle obesity, doctors urge UK government. *Br med J* 2014; 348: 3; C Smyth. Breathe out to shed the pounds. *Times, Lond* 2014; December 17: 7.

3   K Lay. Obese suffer anti-fat bias from NHS. *Ibid* 2017; April 11: 16; O Moody. Loneliness worse for teenagers' health than taking no exercise. *Ibid* 2016; January 5: 29; C Smyth. Live longer in 'healthy towns': NHS will design new housing to fight obesity and improve elderly care. *Ibid* 2016; March 1: 1,4; C Smyth. Living by a busy road 'as bad as being overweight'. *Ibid* 2016; October 25: 19; A Nicholls. 'Live longer' towns. *Ibid* 2016; March 3: 28; S-K Templeton. Mind over munch: call to give obese NHS therapy. *Sunday Times, Lond* 2015; November 8: 27.

4   K Lay. Internet diet 'miracles' can be deadly, warns watchdog. *Times, Lond* 2015; December 30: 4; D Sheridan. Food fraud gangsters rake in £1 bn a year *Ibid* 2016; March 25: 35.

5   C Smyth. Trendy desk health claims don't stand up to scrutiny. *Ibid* 2016; March 17: 13.

6   O Moody. Green tea with every meal helps weight-loss. *Ibid* 2015; July 31: 15; M Porter. Our coffee shop habit is piling on the pounds. *Ibid* 2016; May 19: 26.

7   C Smyth. How to fight the flab: avoid TV, diets and coffee shops. *Ibid* 2015; March 13: 8; P Cunliffe. High-tech help to tackle childhood obesity and cut teachers' red tape. *Ibid* 2016; August 24: 39.

8   O Moody. Want to lose weight? Sit quietly and listen to yourself

chewing. *Ibid* 2016; March 17: 14.

9   M Savage. Sweet-makers warn of plain packet fears. *Ibid* 2014; July 25: 6.

10 N Fildes. Smart belt that knows when you've had second helpings. *Ibid* 2015; January 6: 19; C Smyth. 'Patronising' campaign on middle-aged spread ridiculed. *Ibid* 2016; March 7: 6.

11 V Forster. Chew the fat away with bite monitor. *Ibid* 2014; August 13: 4; Anonymous. Sweets on the brain? Blame your internal calorie counter. *Ibid* 2014; October 21: 15; O Moody. 'Smart' plate can count the calories you're about to eat. *Ibid* 2015; May 16: 17; K Lay. Scan your dinner for an instant calorie count. *Ibid* 2016; January 11: 15; A Bryce. Portable DNA kit will reveal what's really in your dinner. *Ibid* 2016; April 11: 17.

12 C Smyth. Academics find smaller plates hold less food. *Ibid* 2015; December 3: 3.

13 N Badshah. Jab brings hope of cure for obesity. *Ibid* 2015; August 20: 19.

14 H Devlin. Turn down the heat and lose weight. *Ibid* 2014; January 23: 12; O Moody. Want to watch your weight? Try a mirror in the dining room. *Ibid* 2015; December 24: 23; T Whipple. Sunbathing stops you gaining weight (well, it works for mice). *Ibid* 2014; October 24: 31; P Bee. Slow down: why eating too quickly is making you fat. *Times, Lond* 2017; November 18: 7. (*See also*: T Whipple. Office air conditioning makes you fat. *Ibid* 2017; April 27: 3.)

15 J Starkey. Kenyan troops run $400m sugar scam. *Ibid* 2015; November 13: 43.

CHAPTER 14:

Alternative (artificial) sweeteners

For those with a 'sweet-tooth' there is always of course the option of using an *artificial* sweetener as a substitute for *refined-sugar*. A sugar substitute is, by definition, a *food additive* which, as far as taste is concerned, resembles the *sweetness* in sucrose/*fructose*. A few are far sweeter than sucrose/*fructose* on a weight-for-weight basis, but possess negligible energy and/or vitamin content. Some are basically *natural* products, while others are entirely *artificial* and *not* related to dietary components.

The ancient *Greek* philosopher – Xenophanes (c.570–476 BC) – is recorded as having 2,500 years ago pronounced that 'If the gods had *not* made golden honey (*see* Chapter 5) we would think that figs were much sweeter than they really are! Hence, artificial sweeteners are arguably overused because they are merely paying obedience to the '*sweet tooth*' of modern *Homo sapiens*![1] This results in children, in particular, abandoning fruit because it is *not* sufficiently sweet. In addition, both could *increase* risk of *type-2-diabetes mellitus* (*see* below). Nevertheless, sugar alternatives are widely used in food products today, especially in the USA, and like everything else about America (good or bad), they will soon be increasingly used in Britain where their market is already apparently worth £66 million per year. Furthermore over one quarter of British households already purchase them![2]

Sorbitol and *xylitol* are examples of fundamentally *natural* sweeteners – some present in berries, fruit, vegetables and mushrooms; however, owing to the fact that it is not commercially profitable to extract them from fruits and/or vegetables, they are produced by catalytic hydrogenation of an appropriate reducing sugar, *eg*, *xylose* is converted to *xylitol*, *lactose* to *lacitol*, and *glucose* to *sorbitol*.

Some benefits are:

- assistance with weight-loss, by replacing *'refined-sugar'* in dietary items,
- *dental care*: non-sugar sweeteners are *not* fermented by oral microflora (mostly bacteria) and thus caries are significantly diminished (*see* Chapter 10),
- in sufferers of *diabetes mellitus* (*see* Chapter 11), in whom regulation of blood-glucose concentration is rendered easier and more straightforward (*see* below),
- prevention of reactive hypoglycaemia during treatment of *diabetes mellitus*; rapid absorption of the glucose moiety of sucrose into the circulation can cause excessive insulin-release with resultant hypoglycaemia,
- in avoidance of processed foods containing *'refined-sugar'*, and
- cost: sugar-substitutes are often (but *not* always) cheaper than *'refined-sugar'*.

Recent evidence suggests that food additives ('emulsifiers' are added to various foodstuffs, including ones to provide sweetness, such as ice cream and chocolate), by changing bacterial flora in the human colon could in themselves cause or be one of the potential causes of obesity. This might explain why obesity-rates in *industrialised* countries all surged simultaneously in the 1980s.[3]

Sugar substitutes do not stimulate insulin-release. Should insulin play a significant rôle in obesity (far from proven), this would be avoided by sugar substitutes! Occasionally, a 'sweet taste', in itself induces an insulin-response.

The *food-industry* is increasingly (in most cases only partly) replacing *'refined-sugar'* by artificial sweeteners, *aspartame* (*see* below) being most widely used; however, *sucralose* (*see* below) is currently becoming cheaper and might subsequently replace it as an alternative. Commonly consumed dietary items containing 'alternatives' are: cereals, diet sodas, and 'sugar-free' desserts (*eg,* ice-cream). Also with their low or non-calorie content; they are frequently used in advertising, especially directed at sufferers from *type-2-diabetes*. *Xylitol* and *saccharin* are of course *not* associated with dental caries (*see* Chapter 10).

Historical use

Pursuit of an *artificial sweetener* is by no means a *new* quest (*see* above); and inhabitants of ancient Rome felt that they had detected one! They boiled grape juice in lead pots to produce a sugar-syrup concentrate – *sapa*. Like other lead salts the acetate has a sweet taste – utilised by them in sweetening wine. Lead acetate from pots was however a *toxic* component, culminating in lead poisoning. Substantial evidence suggests that Pope Clement II (1005–47) died from effects of lead, and it is possible that Ludwig van Beethoven (1770–1827) too might have died of lead poisoning resulting from wine adulterated with this element. Use of sweeteners thus dates from the days of ancient Rome, but since *modern* introduction – beginning with saccharin in 1897 – there have not surprisingly been serious alarms concerning *toxicity*, and they are currently present in numerous products ranging from drinks, desserts and junk food (*see* above), to cakes, chewing gum and toothpaste. An ongoing problem is that the more they are consumed, frequently unknowingly, the greater an innate craving for sweet food becomes, which in itself encourages obesity, glucose intolerance, and the major complication of obesity – *type-2-diabetes*.[4] But their use in individuals suffering from *diabetes* is clearly valuable. Although most are probably entirely safe, the suspicion persists that they *might* stimulate appetite and thus themselves *contribute* to obesity! Also, possible *carcinogenicity* is an ever present concern. Overall however, artificial sweeteners have the propensity to prevent excessive weight-deposition and obesity, and also avoidance of dental decay, as well as prevention of *diabetes mellitus*.

Lead acetate is a salt of acetic acid which, despite serious side-effects was, as we have seen, used as a sweetener in ancient Rome (*see* above). This had probably been the *first* 'alternative' sweetener. In ancient Rome honey was of course available as a sweetener, but it was apparently in short supply. However, grapes were plentiful and by boiling these unfermented fruits for long periods, it was possible to produce a sweet liquid (lead acetate). Some historians have, in fact, even attributed this to the 'fall of the Roman Empire'!

Examples of 'alternative' sweeteners
Recent attempts to produce *lead acetate* as a sweetener have completely failed to remove *all* lead. Artificial sweeteners in common use today,

arranged in order of approximate sweetness compared to that of refined sucrose are:

Sucralose which is heat stable, non-calorie, and is *320* to *1,000* times as sweet as sucrose, twice that of saccharin, and three times that of *aspartame*. Discovered by Tate & Lyle scientists and researchers at Queen Elizabeth College, London in 1976, it is probably the *safest* artificial sweetener currently available, despite the fact that fears of leukaemia in rats were raised in 2013.

Approximately *400* times sweeter than sucrose is **saccharin,** which was first produced at Johns Hopkins University, USA in 1897; it is widely used in drinks, sweets, medicines, and toothpaste. *Saccharin* has the disadvantage of being unstable when heated, but nevertheless stores well. A cyclamate/saccharin combination (10: 1) is widely used in those countries which legally allow its use, and it is occasionally used with *aspartame*. *Saccharin* may trigger insulin production in both humans and rats, and is widely used in western countries despite concern about an association with bladder neoplasia in rats.

The **mogrosides** are a group of chemical compounds originating with a glycoside derived from certain plants, *eg,* fruit of the gourd vine – *Luo han guo (Siraitia grosvenori).* Some are natural sweeteners *300–400* times sweeter than sucrose, and have been used since 2013 in *natural* sweetener products available in Australia.

Aspartame is an artificial, non-saccharide sweetener. It was first synthesised by J M Schlatter a chemist working for the US firm, Searle and Co in 1965. It is about *200* times sweeter than sucrose but with a calorific value approaching zero. *Aspartame* is probably the most controversial of widely-used artificial sweeteners, being hydrolysed in the small-intestine into aspartic acid, phenylalanine and methanol. Despite several side-effects, it has been declared safe for human use by some 90 countries provided consumption is at current levels. However, in April 2015, unlike in the UK, it was declared unhealthy in the USA, and in consequence excluded from *Diet Pepsi*. *Aspartame* has also been associated with numerous side-effects, some possessing a genetic basis; headache seems the most common undesirable one, and although a carcinogenic effect has been suggested, there is apparently no good evidence for this. Owing to production of phenylalanine it is, of course, contraindicated in those suffering from phenylketonuria (PKU). An article in *Applied Physiology, Nutrition and Metabolism* has indicated that in mice, aspartame can cause hyperglycaemia and weight gain.[5]

Acesulfame potassium is a calorie-free artificial sweetener discovered accidentally in 1967 by a K Clauss and H Jensen in Germany. It is *200* times as sweet as sucrose, and one third that of *sucralose*. Heat-stable, it is often used in association with another sweetener. Suspicions continue about possible carcinogenicity, although the *Food and Drug Administration* (FDA) has approved its use in the USA.

Stevia is another sweetener or 'sugar substitute' consisting of an extract from plant leaves of *Stevia rebaudiana* – native to South America. It is a glycoside, heat-stable and non-fermentable – with only a negligible effect on blood glucose. *Stevia* has been used for many hundreds of years in Brazil and Paraguay and for several decades in Japan. The active component possesses up to *150* times the sweetness of sucrose. *Stevia* contains virtually no calories, does not raise blood glucose and is heat-stable; it is thus used in baking.[6] Owing to the fact that both cyclamate (and saccharin) were suspected of being carcinogenic in the 1970s, *stevia* was cultivated only in Japan for use as a sweetener. It became popular in the USA in the 1980s, although its use remains illegal in some countries.

Sodium cyclamate is an artificial sweetener *30–50* times sweeter than sucrose, and was discovered in 1937 at the University of Illinois. Relatively inexpensive compared with other sweeteners, it is stable when heated. *Cyclamate* is frequently used with other sweeteners, *eg*, ten parts of *cyclamate* to one of *saccharin*. This sodium or calcium salt of cyclamic acid has had a chequered history, having been banned by the FDA in 1970 owing to the fact that when combined with *saccharin*, it was occasionally responsible for bladder carcinoma in rats when used over long periods. *Cyclamate* is now widely used (apart from the USA) as a sweetener.

Xylitol is a sugar alcohol; although approximately as sweet as sucrose, it possesses 33% fewer calories, and has the advantage, unlike sucrose, of being responsible for few dental caries. Xylitol was discovered in the very late *nineteenth* century by German and French chemists, and as a safe sweetener, without toxicity or carcinogenicity,[7] was popularised in European countries. It is present in fibres of numerous fruits and vegetables, and can also be extracted from various berries, oats, mushrooms, corn husks, sugar-cane bagasse and birch. It is used in: chewing gum, lozenges and nasal sprays. Like *sorbitol*, xylitol is *not* absorbed from the gastro-intestinal tract, and thus passes into the colon unaltered, where it is a substrate for bacteria with production of both gas and water – consequently having a laxative effect.[8] Studies in Finland in the 1970s suggested, but failed to prove, that it is 'tooth friendly' (*see* Chapter 10). *Xylitol* is however toxic, and possibly life-threatening to dogs!

Sorbitol (glucitol) is a sugar-alcohol which is slowly metabolised in the human body; it is approximately 60% sweeter than sucrose. It occurs naturally in numerous fruits and berries in trees belonging to the *Sorbus* genus. Discovered in 1872 in fresh juice of mountain berries, it is present in apples, plums, pears, cherries, dates, peaches and apricots. *Sorbitol* is a frequent component of 'sugar-free' chewing gum. It also contains approximately half the calorie value of sucrose, and is of value in management of diabetes.

In the campaign to reduce dietary '*refined-sugar*' (to which this book is largely devoted) artificial sweeteners might constitute a substitute in some foods; however, some studies suggest that they themselves promote weight-gain, primarily because they do *not* send 'satiety' messages (*via leptin*) to the hypothalamus (*see* Chapter 9). Also, they might give rise to difficulty in ensuring that different products have similar degrees of sweetness – important if some palates have adjusted to reduced sweetness.

Undesirable side-effects of 'sweeteners'

A word of *caution* in the use of sweeteners is however required, because experiments in mice with *saccharin, sucralose* and *aspartame* – which as this chapter has recorded, are often many times sweeter than '*refined-sugar*', but provide *no* calories – have revealed development of glucose *intolerance* in animals – which they are intended to prevent. Whether that observation, as well as weight-gain', also applies to *H sapiens* remains unclear, but is denied by certain drink manufacturers. A suggested mechanism for this effect is by alteration of composition and range of colonic flora; the '*new*' bacteria being ones previously associated with obesity! The sum total is that some sweeteners *might* contribute to the *type-2-diabetes* epidemic which they were intended to prevent. This study was carried out at the *Weizmann Institute,* published in *Nature,* and was also reported in the London *Times* newspaper.[9]

Another side-effect indicates that *female* fertility might be impaired by some additives; this concern results from a large study at Sao Paulo, Brazil in which women receiving IVF treatment were far less likely to conceive while receiving artificial sweeteners.[10] On another tack, artificial sweeteners have recently been incorporated into children's meals in order to reduce unacceptable ingredients, including '*refined-sugar*'. Is this wise? They might in fact *increase* the incidence of diabetes in later life![11]

So commonly are artificial sweeteners used in Britain today that the term is widely used in everyday life, like so many others, *not* always in its original context.[12]

In **conclusion**, the best overall advice must be to reduce both consumption of '*refined-sugar*' *and* also that of artificial sweeteners, and to concentrate instead on more healthy foodstuffs, including more fruit and vegetables.

References and notes

1   O Moody. Food companies urged to cut sweeteners. *Times, Lond* 2016; June 11: 4. (*See also*: note 8 below.)

2   A Epstein. Artificial sweeteners: what you need to know: aspartame has been dropped from Diet Pepsi in the US due to bad press. So how safe are sweeteners? *Times 2, Lond* 2015; May 2: 6; Anonymous. *British Pharmacopoeia* London; HM Stationery Office 2016.

3   J Leake. Food additive linked to obesity. *Sunday Times, Lond* 2016; January 31: 19; J Ungoed-Thomas. It's a bitter blow – low calorie sweeteners may fatten us up. *Ibid* 2017; January 8: 8.

4   Op cit. *See* notes 1 and 2 above.

5   *Ibid*; Anonymous. Sweetener causes mice health issues. *New Scientist* 2016; 3 December: 16.

6   Op cit. *See* note 2 above.

7   *Ibid*.

8   Anonymous. Sugary challenge. *New Scientist* 2014; January 18: 4.

9   H Thomson. Sweeteners linked to glucose intolerance: world's most popular food additives are back in the spotlight. *Ibid* 2014; 20 Sept: 8–9. T Whipple. Sweeteners linked to increased risk of diabetes. *Times, Lond* 2016; May 26: 18. (*See also*: H Devlin. Doubts over safety of sweeteners. *Ibid* 2014; September 18: 17; Anonymous. Artificial sweeteners are linked to raised risk of diabetes. *Ibid* 2017; September 14: 22.

10 O Moody. Artificial sweeteners can reduce fertility. *Ibid* 2016; October 17: 1, 2; J Ungoed-Thomas. Child food guru stirs in additives. *Sunday Times, Lond* 2015; April 26: 8.

11 A Lively. Artificial sweeteners: A L Kennedy's new novel is just too nice for its own good. *Ibid (Culture)* 2016; May 15 (A review of a new novel by A L Kennedy); Op cit. *see* note 2 above.

CHAPTER 15:

Surgical management of obesity

Clearly, surgery for obesity is a 'last resort' line of management – after all alternative *medical* procedures have failed. Surgery for *extreme* obesity had its origin(s) in the late 1960's – at a time when favoured operations were: *vertical banded gastroplasty* and *gastric stapling* – neither of which is commonly used today. Technically known as *bariatric* surgery this strategy has two major targets:

- reduction of food intake – by limiting stomach capacity, and
- lessening digestion and absorption – by restriction of the absorptive area of the small intestine (*ie*, short bowel syndrome).

The object is to reduce incidence of both *morbid obesity* and *associated complications*, *eg, type-2-diabetes mellitus* [DM], vascular disease, ischaemic cardiac disease [ICD] and stroke, respiratory problems (especially sleep apnoea), joint/back pain, urinary incontinence, peripheral vascular problems, menstrual irregularity, and certain types of headache, with the obvious intention of reducing potential for further weight-gain. Complications resulting from *severe* obesity in the series reported below were:

- Type-2-diabetes – 28%,
- Major depression – 7%,
- Coronary artery disease – 14–19%, and
- Osteoarthritis – 10–17%

Original *indications* – in the 1960s – were:

- >100lb (45kg) above ideal body weight, and
- >80lb (36 kg) above ideal body weight when accompanied by significant complications.

The *raison d'être* for bariatric surgery in obesity is thus principally to reduce weight, induce remission of obesity-related disease and its complications, and consequently to improve overall quality of life.

Indication for surgery is *currently* usually the *Body Mass Index* (BMI) of >40 kg.m^{-2}. However, recent guidelines suggest one of >35 kg.m^{-2} when associated with significant complications and might be more relevant. There is now increasing concern also that *surgery* based on BMI alone is probably incorrect. Individuals of 'Asian origin' with a BMI which is lower 'could be considered' owing to the fact that they are unduly 'vulnerable to *diabetic* complications'. The British government's health watchdog is currently seeking a superior replacement for BMI (*see* above); a new measure of obesity (instigated by the *National Institute for Health and Care Excellence* [NICE]) focusing upon the waist/height ratio – which it is estimated will reclassify an additional seven million individuals as obese. It is apparently anticipated that women will be most affected by this modification.[1]

Surgical procedures

There are currently three major categories of accepted surgical procedure:

- **Restrictive**: Vertical band gastroplasty,
  Adjustable gastric band,
  Sleeve gastrectomy,
  Intragastric balloon (gastric balloon), and
  Gastric plication
- **Malabsorptive**: Biliopancreatic diversion
  Jejunoileal bypass, and
  Endoluminal sleeve
- **Mixed**: Gastric bypass
  Sleeve gastrectomy with duodenal switch, and
  Implantable gastric stimulation

'Restrictive' procedures leave the gastrointestinal tract essentially unaltered, and as a consequence risks of metabolic complications are minimal. Details of the five surgical operations under this heading include:

- *Vertical banded gastroplasty* – in which part of the stomach is permanently stapled, thus reducing gastric size,
- *Adjustable Gastric Band* ('Lap Band') – in which capacity of the stomach is merely reduced with a silicone band; this has the advantage that it can be performed laparoscopically, and has a very low mortality rate – 0.05%,
- *Sleeve Gastrectomy* – in which the stomach is greatly reduced from its original size to about 15%. Although this procedure has the advantage of removing that portion of the stomach which produces *ghrelin* (the *hormone* which stimulates hunger – *see* Chapter 9); it is *not* however reversible,
- *Intragastric Balloon* – this operation reduces gastric capacity – the balloon can be left *in situ* for up to six months, and
- *Gastric Plication* – this is a version of the more popular gastric sleeve or gastrectomy (*see* above), the sleeve being produced by *suturing* rather than *removal* of gastric tissue.

'Malabsorptive' operations include:

- *Biliopancreatic diversion* (a complex operation – now rarely performed, it having been largely replaced by duodenal switch (*see* below). A smaller stomach is thereby created, and the distal small intestine is connected to the resultant pouch, thus bypassing both duodenum and jejunum. Malabsorptive consequences can be severe, and mineral and vitamin replacement (*see* below) are both imperative. Gallstones are a frequent complication, and cholecystectomy is consequently frequently carried out during the operation.

Both jejunoileal *bypass* and endoluminal *sleeve* operations are now rarely carried out.

'Mixed' operations comprise:
- *Gastric bypass* (Roux-en-y) – this is currently a very popular operation. A small stomach pouch is created with a staple device, and connected to the *distal* small intestine, the upper

small intestine being reattached in a Y-shaped configuration. It is partly reversible, especially when the *dumping syndrome* is a serious complication,

- *Sleeve Gastrectomy with Duodenal Switch* – in which part of the stomach is resected, disconnected from the duodenum, and connected to the distal small intestine. This is a variation of *biliopancreatic diversion – see* above), and
- *Implantable Gastric Stimulation* – in which an electrical device – comparable to a cardiac pacemaker – is implanted by a surgeon. This modifies the enteric nervous system of the stomach, thus giving a false sense of satiety).

How effective are these various operations in weight reduction?
The procedures, together with a recent assessment of their outcome, and published in the *British Medical Journal*, has attempted to answer questions in a large series of USA cases:

Ready communication between the regular physician, and the surgeon undertaking the procedure is essential from the outset:

- every option should first be considered,
- possible outcome of surgery must be fully discussed, and
- requirement for lifelong medical surveillance should be thoroughly and fully explained.

Bariatric surgery as presently applied has been outlined by a group of health-workers at Seattle, USA. Patients considered for operation were: (i) those who had *not* responded successfully to medical management, and (ii) individuals with a BMI >40, or one of >35 in the presence of a 'serious complication of obesity'. Most commonly performed procedures (approximate percentages) were:

- Roux-en-y gastric bypass – 46.6%,
- Vertical sleeve gastrectomy – 27.8%,
- Adjustable gastric banding – 17.8%, and
- Biliopancreatic diversion, with duodenal switch – 22%.

*Type of bariatric procedure applied (*see above*)*
A US group has described the *history* of the various procedures. Although presently based largely on an *anatomical* delineation, it is anticipated that *physiological* ones will ultimately come to the fore. Initially, the proximal jejunum was bypassed, food being directly passed into the *distal* ileum. Although this resulted in dramatic weight-loss, it was abandoned, largely because severe protein-energy malnutrition (adult marasmus) was a frequent result. This procedure was overtaken by either *horizontal gastroplasty* or *vertical banded gastroplasty* – both *restrictive* operations. However, weight re-gain, and/or severe gastro-oesophageal reflux frequently resulted.

In 1969, *gastric bypass* was introduced, and this procedure was later modified into the *Roux-en-y gastric bypass* in order to avoid biliary reflux. *Gastric banding* followed, which later became modified into an adjustable form. Next, an extreme intestinal-bypass was perfected with *biliopancreatic diversion*, with or without distal gastrectomy. Finally, *vertical-sleeve gastrectomy* – which involves a 70% vertical gastric resection – has currently assumed considerable popularity.

Most procedures involve disturbances of *ghrelin, leptin, glucagon-like peptide-1, cholecystokinin, peptide 99*, as well as intestinal microbiology, and bile acids; in future these will achieve greater prominence than strictly *anatomical* considerations.

Countries which had performed >10,000 operations in 2011 were:

- USA and Canada – 101,645 interventions,
- Brazil – 65,000,
- France – 27,648,
- Mexico – 19,000,
- Australia and New Zealand – 12,000, and
- UK – approximately 10,000.

Complications of bariatric surgery
Incidence of complications in this US study during the initial 30–180 post-operative days varied from four to 25%. Post-operative mortality is normally low (<0.3%), and was rarely as high as 20%. Some have been accompanied by a higher complication rate: pulmonary complications,

vomiting, wound infection, haemorrhage, and/or anastomotic leak. Many however have incorporated older techniques (*see* above), and mortality-rate in them was as low as 0.25%.

In the long-term, the most common adverse effects were: iron-deficiency anaemia (as high as 15%); vitamin and mineral deficiency, and reduction in calcium, vitamin D, zinc and copper – which were common. In addition, psycho-social risks (including suicide) should *not* be underestimated.

The authors of this north American *review* concluded that although *short-term* results of *bariatric* surgery were extremely encouraging, *long-term* ones were impossible to evaluate at present, because the procedures had only been in place for a relatively short time. Complications should not however be underestimated, and both short and long-term risks (including suicide) should all be taken into account. Above all, it should be stressed that thorough explanation, which *must* involve both physician and surgeon, is *essential*.[2]

The situation in Britain

Because obesity is more common, and consequently *bariatric* surgery in particular has been developed to a greater extent in the USA, much of this chapter has concentrated on experience there. However, with obesity now also escalating in the UK, this form of management has recently undergone, and will undoubtedly attain, far greater prominence.

Criteria for surgery approved by the *National Institute for Clinical Excellence* (NICE) are a BMI of >40, or if significant complications exist, 35.[3] Recently, several pleas for more widespread application of *bariatric* surgery, especially when obesity is accompanied by a complication – *diabetes mellitus* in particular – have been aired in Britain.[4] One proviso was that in those who are 'too overweight', surgery simply will not work – the major reason being that an associated factor such as smoking renders such patients an unacceptable health risk.[5] A further problem is that numerous layers of fat and sheer weight of the obese patient is too great for many surgeons, and imposes an excessive strain; therefore robots are being used to lighten the load![6]

Bariatric surgery in Britain has in fact become a highly topical matter because it can now be carried out *free* under the *National Health Service*

(NHS), the principal *raison d'être* of this offer being to reduce the extent of the current *type-2-diabetes epidemic*, as well as other serious complications of obesity which are costing the NHS astronomical sums of money.[7] Not surprisingly the announcement by NICE met with a great deal of hostility from individuals who consider that in the first place individuals should not have allowed themselves to have become grossly overweight, but also that obese people should reduce weight by *orthodox* methods.[8] Intention to offer increased quantities of *free* surgery was also strongly criticised by psychiatrists for the reason that this does *not* correct the underlying 'eating disorder' resulting in obesity; as a result patients either become depressed, or in many cases turn to alcohol.[9] Although one million people were expected to be offered surgery, a subsequent article in the *Times* newspaper had serious doubts about this number. Not all obese individuals opt for surgery, other methods of weight-reduction including a healthier lifestyle being favoured by many, while general practitioners also frequently deny access to *bariatric* surgery.[10]

However, between 2011 and 13, 'hundreds [of individuals] under the age of 25' in Britain had apparently been subjected to surgery. Many had lost a significant proportion – up to 60% – of 'excess weight', while two-thirds had undergone total reversal of *type-2-diabetes*. It was therefore concluded that the procedure was overall worthwhile as a money-saving strategy for the NHS.

PRIMARY CARE AFTER *BARIATRIC*, OR 'WEIGHT-LOSS' SURGERY

There are several criteria which should be stressed in *primary care management* following weight-loss surgery. These were dealt with in depth in a BMJ article in 2016:

- During the first 30 post-operative days, severe abdominal pain, tachycardia, pyrexia, chest pain, dyspnoea and continuous vomiting can be encountered. All of these warrant emergency referral,
- Monitoring of cardiovascular disease, and a known complication (*eg, diabetes*) is essential, and
- Life-long supplementation with vitamins and minerals is required.[11]

A FAMOUS EXAMPLE OF BARIATRIC SURGERY

As a high-profile example of this operation strategy, *bariatric* surgery, was performed on a previously extremely fit and healthy football (soccer) player. In 2015, the 55-year-old world-famous footballer, *Diego Maradona* (1960–present) underwent *gastric bypass* surgery with an intention of losing 12-stone. This was apparently the *second* time he had been subjected to surgery for 'ballooning weight'![12]

General surgery

A decision by the NHS to ban support for general surgery in individuals who are both obese and in addition tobacco *smokers*, is also open to criticism. It is also simply wrong to deny surgery in general because research has apparently indicated that fat patients have as good a chance as thin ones of recovery *after* weight-loss. Surgical operations are apparently also more successful when the relevant individual has undergone a period of dieting prior to surgery. As a general rule, it should be noted that being overweight increases the risk of any surgical operation. So 'hard-up' is the NHS, that *smokers* and those who are overweight are already facing difficulties obtaining a *general* surgical procedure.[13]

Transplant surgery

Although not directly connected with *bariatric* surgery, a recent article indicating that *transplant* surgery could be compromised by obese *donors* is of serious concern. This is a somewhat unexpected and until now an unreported corollary of obesity which has only recently received attention. As transplant donors become older (over a third are apparently now > 60 years), the proportion of overweight individuals has clearly escalated, and in consequence donors of a kidney, liver or heart are considerably less satisfactory to *transplant* surgeons. As a result, 'unhealthy' organs are increasingly being used because waiting for a more suitable donor is becoming increasingly risky.[14]

References and notes

1   N Hellen. BMI gives false hope to '7m overweight'. *Sunday Times, Lond* 2015: June 21: 11; P Cordero, JLI, JA Oben. Bariatric surgery as a treatment for metabolic syndrome. *J R Coll Phys Edinb* 2017; 47: 364–8.

2   D E Arterburn, A P Courcoulas. Bariatric surgery for obesity and metabolic conditions in adults. *Br med J* 2014; 349 (September 20): 28–32.

3   A Fiennes. Bariatric surgery – belief, biology or behaviour. *Trans Med Soc Lond* 2014–14.; 130: 123–9; C Smyth. Obese must explain why they deserve weight-loss surgery. *Times, Lond* 2017; October 9: 12.

4   Anonymous. Scalpel please: gastric surgery can achieve extraordinary results for diabetes sufferers. *Ibid* 2016; May 25: 27; C Smyth. Million people should be given weight-loss surgery. *Ibid* 2015: December 23: 12; R Welbourne, *et al*. Bariatric surgery: the UK should do more. *Br med J* 2016; 353 (May 14): 263–5; C Smyth. Gastric band in a pill provides quick fix for ballooning weight. *Times, Lond* 2017; May 18: 4.

5   J Hickson. Obesity problem. *Ibid* 2014; July 14: 27; A Doyle. Surgery won't work for patients who are too overweight. *Ibid* 2016; April 22: 26.

6   J Leake, S Mararike. Robots lighten load of surgery on obese. *Sunday Times, Lond* 2016; April 17: 11.

7   G Swerling. Doctors attack quick-fix plan for more gastric bands to fight obesity. *Times, Lond* 2015: January 5: 4; C Smyth. Obese will get free surgery on the NHS: up to one million could qualify for treatment. *Ibid* 2014; July 11: 1, 4; K Lay. Weight-loss surgery can cut diabetes risk. *Ibid* 2014; November 3: 9; C Smyth. Young people join rush for 'good value' weight-loss surgery. *Ibid* 2014; November 10: 18; C Smyth. Two million could get NHS weight-loss surgery. *Ibid* 2014; November 27: 5; J Wise. NICE advice on obesity could mean 5000 more operations a year. *Br med J* 2014; 349 (November 29): 1.

8   O Kamm. More surgery for the obese is a waste of precious money. *Times, Lond* 2014; November 27: 34; T Allen-Mills. Tubby town says no to surgery, yes to exercise. *Sunday Times, Lond* 2014; November

30: 21.

9   Op cit. *See* note 7 (Smyth, November 10 2014) above.

10 Z Kmietowicz. GP commissioning failures deny obese patients access to surgery. *Br med J* 2014; 348 (January 11): 3.

11 M Moore, J Hopkins, P Wainwright. Primary care management of patients after weight-loss surgery. *Br med J* 2016; 352 (March 12): 406–11.

12 J Hider. Maradona goes under the knife to lose 12 stone *Times, Lond* 2015; November 18: 41.

13 C Smyth. Surgery 'rationing' for the obese and smokers. *Ibid* 2015; March 7: 16; S-K Templeton. NHS units impose surgery ban on obese and smokers. *Sunday Times, Lond*: July 23: 4; C Smyth. Patients will be ordered to slim down for operations. *Times, Lond* 2015; March 9: 10; K Lay. Weight is not a reason to deny surgery to obese people. *Ibid* 2015; November 30: 19; C Smyth. Obese patients and smokers are denied surgery. *Ibid* 2016; October 7: 10; M Battersby. NHS chiefs ban surgery for obese patients and smokers. *Ibid* 2016; September 3: 37; S-K Templeton, J Ungoed-Thomas. Smokers and obese 'denied treatment by hard-up NHS'. *Sunday Times, Lond* 2016; October 23: 11; K Gibbons. Obese must lose weight or miss out on surgery. *Times, Lond* 2016; November 29: 1,2.

14 C Smyth. Transplants at risk as donors get fatter. *Ibid* 2014; July 9: 8; C Smyth. NHS rations surgery for the obese. *Ibid* 2016; April 22: 19.

Chapter 16:

Lack of intervention by the British government: consumers *versus* the sugar/food industry

By 2013, the simple fact that the majority of the British population, especially infants and children, were consuming far too much *'refined-sugar'*, and that this was contributing to the *obesity epidemic*, was clear. But the British (Conservative) government was still doing *nothing* about it, largely because it did *not* want to upset the food industry.

In early March 2016 the President of UK's *Faculty of Public Health* was joined by the CEO of *Diabetes UK*, the President of the *Royal College of Paediatricians and Child Health*, and the *Royal College of Physicians' Special Adviser on Obesity* in a letter to the London *Times* newspaper, expressing disappointment that 'the government [had] yet again *delayed* publishing its childhood obesity strategy'. In order to be effective, it claimed, 'it must include … targets for manufacturers to make their products healthier, restricting *marketing* of unhealthy food and drinks to children *together with* introduction of a 20% *tax* on sugar-sweetened drinks'. They once again stressed the *urgency* of the matter.[1]

The history of consumption of excessive quantities of *'refined-sugar'* (sucrose) has already been outlined in this book and involves, it should be recalled, a totally 'alien' item in the human diet! *'Refined-sugar'* is now however, a low-priced source of calories and greatly favoured too by sportsmen and women among others. Its *undesirability* is *not* solely due to its high calorific value and ability to *cause* obesity combined with a loss of essential nutrients, but also because it contains a very high concentration of the sweetener – *fructose* (*see* Chapter 8) – which cannot be handled by human metabolic processes which have arguably had insufficient time to evolve appropriately (*see* Chapter 4).

Food industrialists and those supporting the sugar 'lobby' invariably begin with the premise that *sweetness* is *essential* (especially in childhood), and that reinforcement of *'refined-sugar'* with added vitamins etc, which ancestors of present-day *Homo sapiens* obtained from 'natural' dietary sources, is merely of secondary importance.

To what extent should 'refined-sugar' *be restricted?*
Most are therefore agreed that something should urgently be done to solve the UK's *obesity epidemic*; but what? The obvious answer is for the population to consume less food/drink containing *'refined-sugar'*. But that is easier said than done! Many have introduced a *political* dimension (*see* below), while others have likened this to the *tobacco* dilemma and have sought government *legislation* (*see* below). A decline in *'refined-sugar'* intake had been strongly recommended in several reports, including one from the *World Health Organisation* (WHO), and as a result the world price of sugary foods had, by 2013, already slumped.

The first major question to be asked thus surrounded the extent of the recommended reduction in *'refined-sugar'* intake.[2] The *industry* suggested that a reduction in sugar intake to 5% of calories for example, 'could make people even fatter' because it 'could result in a 'higher intake of both fatty and other high-calorie foods'. Despite proposed initiatives, it seemed that nothing could be done in a constructive way before the *food-industry* acted.[3]

Demand for *'refined-sugar'* seemed however at that time to be declining; the *Times* reported for example, in late 2014 that 'a decision in Brussels to dismantle European sugar quotas' had contributed to a glut in the global supply, resulting in a slump by 56% in *Associated British Foods'* sugar profits.[4] Also, the *Royal Society for Public Health England* (PHE) launched an appeal to the *European Union* (EU) to make it 'compulsory for alcoholic drinks to be prominently labelled with nutritional information' including *calorie* content.[5] However, some six months later a report from France indicated that 'Winemakers [had] begun a campaign to *dissuade* the [EU] from enforcing such a ban; they were apparently fearful (like the *food-industry*) that sales would in consequence fall further.[6]

Restrictive campaigns over the previous few years had achieved relative success with respect to *salt* reduction in foodstuffs, and likewise reduction in *cigarette* smoking. It was therefore optimistically envisaged by such bodies as *Action on Sugar* that similar strategies would inevitably lead to diminution in '*refined-sugar*' consumption in food/drinks – especially those targeted at infants and children.[7]

Salt

The underlying premise had been that failure to curtail *salt* consumption in Britain in 2013 was currently costing an annual total of 6,000 lives. Although the strategy to reduce *salt* in food had been initiated in 2003, the then government (largely as a result of [Lord] Lansley's intervention) had temporarily abandoned this scheme with disastrous consequences. In subsequent discussion however, fears were raised that there was still considerable confusion concerning the correct allowance of *salt* in children's diets! Concentrations recommended by manufacturers of children's food remained far too high however, and reflected adult levels. Under a deal with the British government, reduced concentration had resulted in the intake being limited to 15%; this modification is estimated to have saved about 9,000 lives annually. In 2015 however, these targets were abandoned, with an estimated cost in mortality of around 6,000 per year (*see* above). The blame, according to the chairman of *Consensus Action on Salt and Health*, lay with Lansley – former *Secretary for Health* and *Leader of the House of Commons* who indicated that the *Department of Health* was 'on the side of the *food industry* and *not* the consumer'. Therefore, should the industry reduce the concentration of '*refined-sugar*' in food (and drink), for how long would this agreement last! A detailed account of the successful regimen to reduce *salt* content in the British diet recommended by the *Food Standards Agency* and later the *Consensus Action on Salt and Health*, and derailed by government policy was provided by the *British Medical Journal*.[8]

Tobacco

Others called for a campaign analogous to that in reduction of *smoking*, which would inevitably include 'plain packets'; opposition again came from the *food industry* as well as supermarkets who argued that promotion of a 'healthy, active lifestyle' coupled with reduction of fat content was needed, and *not* introduction of plain packets. Another viewpoint was aired in an article in the *Journal of Sports Medicine*, which alleged that 'The food-industry [was] behaving in a way similar to *tobacco* companies in trying to deny that sugar and carbohydrates … are causing [this] surge in obesity …'. Lack of physical activity, it claimed, was *more* important than '*refined-sugar*' intake. Assuming that the industry would *not* increase efforts to reduce the calorific value of the national diet, a sugar *tax* or some other regulatory process might be necessary. This article predicted that 'there would eventually be lawsuits *against* the *food-industry* for a [causative] rôle in obesity'. The Vice-President elect of the *Faculty of Public Health* claimed:

> We no longer allow *tobacco* companies to market cheap *cigarettes* to children; [therefore] our kids now deserve equal protection from the cynical marketing of cheap sugary drinks and junk food.

In a subsequent comparison between this campaign and the *tobacco* saga, Susan Jebb (a government food adviser) highlighted the importance of both surroundings and circumstances regulating sugar intake; *eg,* people are greatly influenced by other individuals performing a similar activity, and will automatically follow suit! As an example: 'If I'm in a meeting and there are biscuits on the table, I'm … likely to eat [one, but] if I'm in my office [alone], I wouldn't go out and search for one.

In the early *sixteenth* century, *tobacco* became popular in 'western' civilisations, although it had probably already been known for up to eight *millennia* in southern America. It was in the 1530s that the French explorer Jacques Cartier (1491–1557) brought its use to western civilisation's attention, and some 30 years later, a French diplomat Jean Nicot (1530–1600) introduced it to the French court. The addictive habit of *tobacco* smoking rapidly diffused across Europe and beyond. In the mid-*eighteenth* century Carolus Linnaeus (1707–78) the botanist, introduced *Nicotina* as the plant's generic name, and after the *addictive* element had been isolated by two Germans in 1828, the plant was known as *nicotine*. To render *tobacco* palatable (in the form used in cigarettes, cigars, pipes and snuff, etc), the leaves of the plant are 'cured' *ie,* parts of the 'chemical cocktail' within the leaves are oxidised and degraded. As late as the *seventeenth* century, the advisability of smoking *tobacco* was sharply divided; King James I (1566–1625), for example, wrote *A Counterblaste to tobacco* (1604), in which he wrote:

> A custome loathsome to the eye, hatefull to the Nose, harmefull to the braine, dangerous to the Lungs, and in the blacke stinking fume thereof, nearest resembling the horrible Stigian smoke of the pit that is bottomelesse.

However, it rapidly became a panacea for all health problems – some organic and others psychological. Only relatively recently (in the 1950s) did the detrimental effects on health and its association with bronchial carcinoma become widely appreciated in Britain. In fact, *tobacco* has, over the centuries, probably killed more than any other plant! It is now bracketed with heroin and cocaine as being highly addictive. Financial rewards were soon (from the *seventeenth* century onwards) reaped on *tobacco*, and they have since been exploited by the *tobacco* industry. As sales have recently declined – resulting from recognition of associated morbidity and mortality – *tobacco* giants in industry have sought means of alternative advertising and other strategies to sell their products. On an experimental tack, *Nicotiana* sp had in the *nineteenth* and early *twentieth* centuries served as a model for plant hybridisation and biology; for example, it became the *first* artificially *genetically modified* plant, thus paving the way for the genetically modified crop revolution.[9]

An early suggestion that publicity on *tobacco* restriction could be applied to tackling the *obesity epidemic* came from Jebb[10]. Although by no means the first, she pointed out the confusion in the public's mind about what constitutes a healthy diet and *cause* of obesity: they were totally unclear at that time for example, about the rôle of dietary fat! Working along Jebb's lines, '*refined-sugar*' was thus termed the '*new*' tobacco. However, Lansley ridiculed that approach (*see* below) before the House of Commons; he was in effect defending the *food industry* against the medical profession, before Parliament!

The point was, that the *tobacco industry*, the food industry and the British government were all supporting '*refined-sugar*' largely because it continued claiming (but it is by no means clear that it believed what it preached) that other factors – such as reduction in exercise – were more important in causing obesity. In fact, so dependent on advertising both in Britain and abroad was the *tobacco* industry (or '*Big Tobacco*'), that it had paid 'huge bribes' in order to protect sales and oppose alternative companies in East Africa – a totally immoral exercise![11]

Parallels with the *tobacco* saga were also highlighted by Peter Sever (of the medical profession) in early 2014; it had taken about *fifty* years to 'control' the *tobacco* industry, which delayed legislation over 'content and marketing … its products'. Will it therefore take *fifty* years, he asked, to 'legislate over the food industry and its high-pressure marketing [of] poor-quality nutritional products …' which combined with lack of exercise is obesity's major cause?[12]

Alcohol

Most individuals associate the stout middle-aged man with a 'beer belly' with an excess of alcohol consumption. Alcohol is therefore – in the minds of most – an important *cause* of obesity. But is this association justified, especially from a *causative* angle? Some have even recommended that to 'cure' obesity, food should be replaced with alcohol! Others claim that the '*calorie*-count' in alcoholic beverages is so high that it must be strictly limited, especially in the overweight. However, the anti-alcohol 'establishment' insists that dangers of alcohol (especially if you are a smoker) are so great that all forms of it should be completely banned. Overall, experience with alcohol (in all its forms) had little to add overall to the campaign to limit '*refined-sugar*', other than to ban it altogether![13]

Thus, experience with *salt*, *tobacco* and *alcohol* had had little to add to the '*refined-sugar*' controversy, other than the government's neglect of the consumer, and clear support for the *food industry*.

An underlying problem concerns independent *experts*

The most serious underlying problem lay in the fact that although the vast majority of organisations advised a *healthy* diet, while many proponents, posing as an *independent* body, were in fact paid by various sections of the *food-industry*.[14] An article published in the London *Sunday Times* newspaper in 2015 made that abundantly clear. The *British Nutrition*

Foundation (BNF), for example, is usually regarded as a thoroughly respectable organisation, the advice of which on ideal dietary components can be trusted; however, like other such organisations it has transpired to be largely dependent on funding derived from the institutionalised food-industry and is concerned primarily with shareholders of manufacturers of food products rather than the interests of the laity (often children, and to a lesser extent their parents) seeking *independent* advice. The following article read:

> Schoolchildren are being taught that foods high in fat or sugar are a necessary part of a *balanced* diet, under guidelines and teaching materials produced by an organisation partly funded by food manufacturers. The [BNF], which includes *Coca-Cola*, *Mars* and *British Sugar* among its members, has helped write 'core competencies' on diet and health for school lessons on nutrition. [A] seven-page document makes [absolutely] *no reference* [my italics] to obesity or … links between foods high in saturated fat and sugar and heart disease and diabetes. In [their] paper, the BNF recommends the use of the government's *'eatwell'* plate – a pictorial representation of … foods that make up a *healthy* diet. One of the groups is 'foods and drinks high in fat and/or sugar', such as cola, cake, crisps, sweets and biscuits.
>
> The government's own material makes clear that these 'are not essential to a healthy diet, and should be consumed only in small amounts'. However, a BNF presentation to support teaching on the *eatwell* plate [fails to] make it clear that foods high in fat or sugar are *not* essential, describing all … different food groups shown on the plate as those 'which are needed to make up a healthy, varied diet'.

Details of the rôle of the BNF in shaping children's lessons on nutrition came *after* … the *life sciences minister* warned that food companies may in future be forced to pay a 'sugar *tax'*. PHE (*Public Health England*) is reviewing the *eatwell* plate, amid demands that cola, sweets and crisps should be removed. It said [that] the BNF disclosed its funding sources, and *its work was* being *reviewed by external experts* [my italics]. The BNF, which produced the guidelines in conjunction with [PHE] says

184

its funding [came] from a variety of sources, including the [*European Union*], and its advice [was] independent. [The] director-general of BNF, said it was clear from other BNF material for teachers that food high in fat and sugar was *not* required for a healthy diet.

A nutritionist said it 'beggared belief' that a can of cola was on the *eatwell* plate and that it was now being embedded in the national curriculum. She emphasised that: '*Advice on nutrition for children needs to be drawn up by experts ... independent of the food industry*' [my italics].

The *Sunday Times* article was followed a week later by a communication from the BNF's *Educational Programme Manager* blaming government for inclusion of *cola*, and adding a *denial* that it 'did *not* single out *cola* as an essential food for health'.[15]

In 2015, the London *Times* newspaper published a prominent article on its front page: '*Fizzy drinks giant pays millions to diet experts: scandal as scientists deny link with obesity*' (*see* fig 16.1). This piece recorded that 'Coca-Cola' had 'poured millions of pounds into British scientific research and healthy-eating initiatives to counter claims that its drinks [were involved in the] *cause* of obesity'.[16]

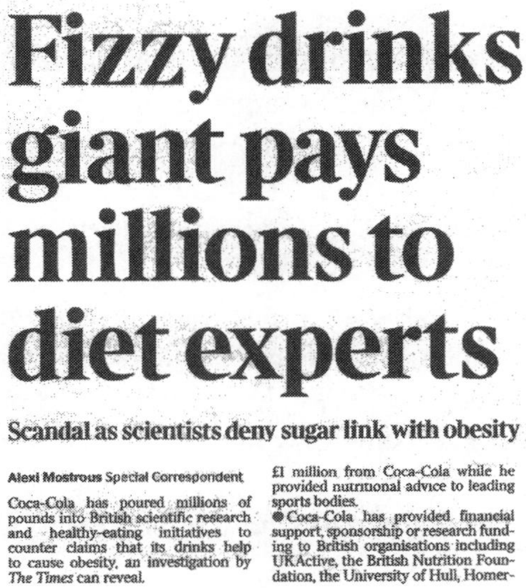

Fizzy drinks giant pays millions to diet experts

Scandal as scientists deny sugar link with obesity

Alexi Mostrous Special Correspondent

Coca-Cola has poured millions of pounds into British scientific research and healthy-eating initiatives to counter claims that its drinks help to cause obesity, an investigation by The Times can reveal.

£1 million from Coca-Cola while he provided nutritional advice to leading sports bodies.

● Coca-Cola has provided financial support, sponsorship or research funding to British organisations including UKActive, the British Nutrition Foundation, the University of Hull, Homer-

Fig 16.1: 2015 headline to an article in London's *Times* newspaper. (*Times, Lond;* October 9: 1, 9.)

In early 2015, the *British Medical Journal* (BMJ) also published results of an investigation to determine to what extent, if any, the country's leading public health experts (*ie,* government-funded organisations, such as the *Scientific Advisory Committee on Nutrition* [SACN] and the [*Medical Research Council*] [MRC]'s *Human Nutrition Research Unit*) were co-operating with the *sugar industry via* research grants, consultancy fees, and other forms of funding. The result of that enquiry was deeply disturbing: 11 bodies it transpired were receiving financial assistance from the food-industry, and in addition at least three government organisations were receiving advice from members supported by the *sugar industry*. Once again, there was clear evidence that instead of working to *improve* the nation's health, the *food industry* was paying 'experts' to make their targets 'respectable' for shareholders.[17]

The SACN (*see* above) had meanwhile confirmed that added sugar should be limited to 5% of an individual's energy intake (*see* above), there being good evidence that some children consume, on average, *three* times that amount. Data from the UK's *National Diet and Nutritional Survey*, for example, indicated that 11–18-year-olds derive 15.6% of their calories from sugar – most in fizzy drinks (*see* above, and Chapter 1), while four to 10-year-olds obtain 14.7% of calories from sugar. Although manufacturers apparently removed 100 billion calories per year, this was less than 6% of the government's target to cut 5 billion calories per day, or 1.8 trillion per year.

What, then, should be done to reduce the overwhelming influence of the sugar industry?

The obvious answer was to find some means of *reducing* overall quantity of '*refined-sugar*' (sucrose) intake throughout the world. In his book, *Pure, White and Deadly* ... Yudkin had addressed the problem of what to do about '*refined-sugar*'; should we:

- leave the onus entirely with the individual, whose health is at risk?
- attempt influence on manufacturers (industrialists) to reduce the amount of 'sugar' in their products? or
- scale down the volume of advertising?

The latter strategy would be comparable to public campaigns against *tobacco* (*see* above), but overall, Yudkin had serious doubts about that approach, which could obviously be applied to the extreme option of banning 'sugar' entirely![18]

In early 2014, the London *Times* newspaper had published an article entitled: ***Sugar is the new tobacco, say doctors***. Written by the newspaper's health correspondent, it advocated reduction in '*refined-sugar*' (sucrose) content of food by a massive 30% within five years, thus reflecting concern of a group of doctors from *Action on Sugar*. This group concluded that: '[This component of diet] has little nutritional value, does *not* make people feel full, and is dangerous beyond merely the number of calories it contains'; it added that the 'sugar we add to food ourselves is dwarfed by the amounts added by food companies'. Furthermore, 'if companies [would] cut down gradually we would all eat 100 calories a day less without noticing [it]'. The group was obviously targeting particularly 'the food and soft drink industry', and it suggested that their plan should be supported by the *Department of Health*. Added comments would focus not solely on obesity, but on *type-2-diabetes*, 'metabolic syndrome', fatty liver, and also alcohol consumption. However, a spokeswoman for the *Food and Drinks Federation* pronounced that:

> Sugars ... consumed as part of a varied and balanced diet are *not* [the] *cause* of obesity; and to this there is no simple or single solution.[19]

The following day, the same newspaper published a further report, also written by its health correspondent, entitled '*Lansley* [*see* above] *ridicules claims that sugar is the new tobacco*'. In this article, in an attempt to defend the *food-industry*, Lansley had evidently told the *House of Commons* (*see* above) 'We have had significant success in the reduction of *salt* in food, but it has to be understood that this can only be achieved [by] working *with* the industry on a *voluntary* basis ... and it can only be done on an incremental basis ... You can't simply slash the sugar in food, otherwise people won't accept it. That is what [the group is] looking for. I don't think it is helped by inaccurate analogies [with *tobacco* restriction] ... *Sugar is an essential component of food* – it's just that sugar *in excess* is inappropriate'. To this, the Chairman of *Action on Sugar* (*see* above) told the reporter that 'Lansley had destroyed a successful policy' on *salt* when he [was] Health Secretary, and he added, 'Frankly, I don't have much time for him. He messed up the [*National Health Service* (NHS)] and ... public health ... [Sugar is] a major source of hidden calories and if you get it down it will help with obesity. [It is] addictive, particularly in young children, and the *food industry* uses it as a weapon to sell rubbish food to young children'.[20]

A major problem with those statements and vehement exchange of views was that the problem was viewed, once again, from the premise that it is *total calories* which matter, rather than a '*toxic*' constituent within '*refined-sugar*'.Above all, however, the *Food Industry* continued with its 'message' that the *cause* of obesity is shrouded in *mystery*, whereas the reality of the situation was that the solution was ... clear, and it is fairly and squarely in their hands. It is not to my mind the *calorie value* of refined sucrose which matters in any case, but its *fructose* component (*see* Chapter 8), which at this high concentration is in consequence totally alien to the human species. '*Refined-sugar*'-containing foods and drinks also *suppress* production of the hormone – *leptin* (*see* Chapter 9) – which transmits the 'message' of *satiety* to the brain – and in consequence inculcates a craving for even more ingested '*refined-sugar*'. The fact is that the *Leader of the House of Commons*, and one suspects the British '*establishment*' is, first and foremost supportive of the *food industry* which is merely exacerbating this disaster, *ie,* an escalating rate of worldwide obesity, and also the frequency of its numerous complications!

Has the human population already become addicted to a high concentration of dietary sucrose?
A major question surrounds the degree of dependence on '*refined-sugar*' to which the world's populations have already been subjected; *ie,* to what extent are we all *addicted* to present levels of '*refined-sugar*' (sucrose) consumption? As pointed out in a subsequent *Times* article, a tendency to be attracted to low-priced offers of sugar-containing products (*see* Chapter 4) has already developed. In a comparison with consumption of low-priced *tobacco* and *alcohol* products, the author of this report highlighted temptation of 'sugar'-containing products, and suggested

that a 30% reduction in the immediate future was unlikely. Furthermore, the writer was dubious that a commodity so much bound up with 'love and giving' will be rapidly discarded, and also the fact that 'sugar' has to some extent filled the gap left by a decline in *tobacco* (and possibly *alcohol*) consumption.[21]

Should legislation *to reduce* 'refined-sugar' *be introduced?* (see also *below*)

Correspondence columns of the *Times* newspaper also emphasised comparison between the present obesity *crisis* and the situation which had recently faced *tobacco* usage. Parallels between *tobacco* consumption and diets high in *saturated fat*, salt and sugars was striking; 'both [were] intensively promoted and marketed by international concerns whose goals were clearly [aimed at] profit-making rather than [promoting] international health'. In the case of *food advertising* however, the most vulnerable members of society – *ie,* children and the 'economically deprived' – were targeted. The aim was 'to give these products health credibility [frequently involving a sporting event] which they simply do not have'. The ultimate solution therefore must lie either with the individual consumer, *or* the *food industry*, but *not* both. A period of about fifty years proved necessary for suitable *legislation* to reduce marketing of *tobacco* products (*see* above); will it therefore take a further half century to introduce suitable *legislation* to modify advertising within the *food industry*?[22]

It was now clear that there was a straightforward battle between what is beneficial to mankind (children in particular) and profits within the *food industry* – who are, after all, in the debate purely to maintain and/ or increase sales! The Chief Executive of *Tesco* apparently admitted that *legislation* 'may [ultimately] be needed' to tackle the obesity problem.[23]

It is perhaps too easy however, to single out the *food-industry* alone for this catastrophe. Media, (including numerous televised cooking programmes), restaurants, schools and parents *too* should clearly take some blame.[24] In this context, it is appropriate to mention repeated attempts by the chef Jamie Oliver to persuade the British government to introduce a 'sugar *tax*'.[25]

Similarity with tobacco and alcohol use (see also *above*)

Enlarging on the close similarity with the *smoking* epidemic (*see* above), the *Times* correspondence column again seems relevant. One letter stressed that *legislation*, rather than illustrations of the disastrous consequences of added sugar was more likely to succeed: what is required is 'an effective strategy' and *not* more useless tactics.[26] Another recommended focusing 'governmental and consumer-led [support for] fresh, locally sourced food sold in local markets'. According to this writer, '[that] will be a quicker [and] more effective way of improving the nation's health than waiting for governments to keep dithering over *legislation* in the face of lobbying from the multinational *food industry*'. It is also worth recalling previous experience with *alcohol* (*see* above): 'Ministers [eventually caved in] to the powerful drinks lobby over plans to impose a *minimum* price for alcohol'. As for *tobacco*, 'plans to introduce plain cigarette packaging in England [were put on hold following] a lobbying campaign by the *tobacco* industry …'.[27]

Further denial of sugar's disastrous effects, by the food industry

In January 2014, the *Times* published a letter from the 'Nutritionist and Nutrition Communications Manager of *Sugar Nutrition UK*'. In this, she pointed out that the WHO's Expert Committee had yet to decide whether or not to issue guidance on reduction of 'sugar' intake (in response to an article in the same newspaper five days previously). More importantly, she indicated that this Committee, as well as the *WHO European Food Safety Authority* and the *UK Department of Health*, had 'reviewed scientific evidence [obtained] over many years and *all* [had] concluded that *the balance of available evidence does* not *implicate sugar in any of the so-called 'lifestyle diseases'* [my italics]'.[28]

Representing the *anti-sugar* side of this debate was *Action on Sugar*, and on the other, the *Food Industry* and the *World Sugar Research Organisation*. Situated between them was the inappropriately-titled *Scientific Advisory Committee on Nutrition* (SACN) (*see* above), consisting of a group of '*independent*' experts advising government; no less than five of this eight-strong delegation transpired to have self-confessed links with the *Food industry*! An Irishman on this Committee – Albert Flynn – claimed for example to have looked closely at a possible link between sugar consumption and obesity for the *European Food Safety Agency* (EFSA), and concluded that 'there was [absolutely] *no* evidence of a "positive correlation" between total sugar intake and obesity'. There was thus overwhelming evidence that decision(s) reached by the advisory meeting held in April 2014 would inevitably be heavily influenced by individuals with links to the sugar industry![29] It is interesting to note again that Yudkin had had personal battles with the *Sugar Industry* which likewise either denied a link with the diseases highlighted by himself, or unjustifiably criticised its research techniques.[30]

By November 2014, it was clear that public feeling was belatedly exerting an impact on the *food-industry*. The *Times* reported in its business section that the *Associated British Foods Industry* had 'suffered a spectacular collapse in sugar profits because of a *worldwide* plunge in the price of this commodity', supply and demand having been regulated by Brussels. In 2012, the industry had in fact been 'churning out … five million tons [of *refined-sugar*] a year' with a corresponding 'half a billion pounds in profits from its [*worldwide*] sugar processing operation'; however, by September 2014, 'sugar profits [had] slumped by 56% from the £189 million' obtained during the previous year (*see* above).[31]

Other views on sugar and obesity
In January 2014, the journal *New Scientist* considered that 'the UK [had] declared war on sugar', thus repeating the nation's partially successful crusade against *salt*. The present strategy, recommended by *Action on Sugar*, it claimed, was to persuade manufacturers to reduce sugar content in food and drink so slowly that consumers would fail to notice it! But it was by *no* means certain that palates would adjust *rapidly*– as they apparently had done with *salt* reduction – to reduced sweetness.[32]

The BMJ again stressed the 'United Kingdom's spiralling obesity crisis' (which was 'more severe than previously thought') and importance of its being brought under control. It recorded that the *National Obesity Forum* (NOF) had 'urged … government to launch harder hitting public health campaigns', and also that more emphasis should be placed on training and incentivising [general practitioners] to have conversations with … patients about their weight' (*see* Chapter 13). Unless something was urgently done', [at least] half of the UK population would be obese by 2050'.[33]

As a result of 63 complaints, a televised *advertising* campaign accompanied by posters claiming that the sports drink *Lucozade Sport* 'hydrates and fuels you better than water', had been banned by the *Advertising Standards Authority*. This also reflected the 'battle over health claims launched by the drinks industry.[34]

Is a 'sugar tax' at last a reality?

A '*sugar-tax*' as a major strategy to reduce '*refined-sugar*' in processed food had of course been suggested on numerous occasions (*see* above), but had repeatedly been repelled by government under continued hounding by the *food industry*. Government had thus been reluctant to act, presumably because its primary intent was to support the *industry*. Not only Jamie Oliver's restaurants (*see* above), but most NHS hospitals had by now imposed their own *sugar taxes*. However, at a time when obesity and perhaps more importantly its complications, were proving so costly to the NHS, one would have thought that this would have been dominant in decisions taken by Britain's rulers.

Whether it was more expedient to impose (i) a '*sugar-tax*' or (ii) legally impose compulsory reduction in the concentration of '*refined-sugar*' were two possible options. The issue therefore posed two potential solutions:

- Ban all '*refined-sugar*' by making it an illegal substance, in a way similar to negotiations on *salt* and *tobacco,* or even by its designation as a dangerous drug, or
- in the event of industry refusing to *reduce* '*refined-sugar*' in food and drink, a *sugar-tax* would be imposed.

On the second tack, complications of obesity were currently costing the NHS so much that according to the *Times*, the UK *Sciences Minister* in May 2015 had given a firm indication that companies selling food causing ill-health would be penalised and its products in consequence *taxed*. He was apparently however, opposed to 'heavy handed' *legislation*.[35]

Taxing drinks which cause obesity and ill-health had of course been recommended by many over several years; a 'sugary drink' *tax* of 20% would significantly reduce the number of obese individuals, the largest fall being in 16–30 year olds who consume far more sugary drinks than older people.[36] Such a scheme would however be (i) difficult to implement, and (ii) not approved by all. Although this in itself could *not* possibly solve the obesity crisis, it would be an effective *public health* measure if implemented in association with other measures (*see* below).[37]

The Chief Medical Officer (CMO) for England – Dame Sally Davies, FRS – had in early 2014 been quoted as declaring her support for a *sugar tax*; she apparently considered that 'Ministers [also] needed to put more pressure on food companies to make ... food in the shops healthier'.[38] In Denmark, a *tax* on saturated *fat* imposed in 2011 had after all reduced demand, increased consumption of both fruit and vegetables, and as a result fewer deaths had occurred. This had however been abolished in late 2012, primarily because the *food-industry* argued strongly against it.[39]

At this stage, it seemed that *legislation* was the sole underlying strategy to reduce obesity, especially in children.[40] There were however two inextricably linked but separate problems before imposition:

- General acceptance that '*refined-sugar*' (sucrose) was itself the *major cause* of obesity, and
- A decision on the magnitude of a '*sugar tax*', and its method of imposition.

Addressing the first problem, the *Times* launched an attack on those 'major food concerns[§§§] which put cash *before* acceptance of the fact that '*refined-sugar*' was a vitally important [factor in causing obesity]'.

> *Coca-Cola* has poured millions of pounds into British scientific research and healthy-eating initiatives to counter claims that its drinks help to cause obesity .... The drinks giant, a major sponsor of the [2016 *Olympic Games*], the *Fifa World Cup* and the *Rugby World Cup*, has financial links to more than a dozen British scientists, including government health advisers and others who cast doubt on the commonly accepted link between *sugary drinks* and the obesity crisis.

[§§§] This report was accompanied by a two-page article by the same author (A Mostrous. How *Coca-Cola* made its friends in the right places : nutrition adviser with ties to the real thing. *Times, Lond* 2015 ; October 9 : 8-9), indicating that '*Coca-Cola*' was, as well as financing several major nutrition organisations, strongly advocating *hydration* in order to sell its products.

Many scientists blame increased sugar consumption for Britain's *obesity epidemic*, which kills up to 53,000 people a year and costs the NHS £5.1 billion annually. A recent report in the *British Journal of Sports Medicine* argued that a poor diet was the prime cause of more disease than physical inactivity, *alcohol* and *smoking* combined.

The full scale of *Coca-Cola* scientific funding can be exposed after the government rejected calls for a *sugar tax* from [among others] the chief medical officer, the *British Medical Association* and [food] celebrities such as Jamie Oliver [*see* above and below].

It can [now] be revealed that:

- *Coca-Cola* spent millions [of pounds] setting up the *European Hydration Institute* [EHI] – an apparently independent research foundation to promote hydration [recommending] that people consume [both] sports and soft drinks of the sort the company sells,
- The chairman of the body's scientific advisory board is a respected professor whose university received almost £1 million from *Coca-Cola* while he provided nutritional advice to leading sports bodies, and
- *Coca-Cola* has provided financial support, sponsorship or research funding to British organisations including *UKActive*, the *British Nutrition Foundation*, the *University of Hull*, *Homerton University Hospital*, the *National Obesity Forum*, *British Dietetic Association*, *Obesity Week 2013* and the *Association for the Study of Obesity*.

In 2013 Spanish researchers had found that scientific papers on *sugary drinks* that were (either) sponsored by or had potential conflicts of interest with the *food and drink industry*, including *Coca-Cola*, were *five times* more likely to find *no link with obesity* than similar papers that were independently funded. They recommended 'special efforts to preclude funding by parties with vested interests at all levels'.

... a board member of the *Faculty of Public Health* wrote: '*Coca-Cola* is trying to manipulate not [only] public opinion but policy and political decisions. Its tactics echo those used by the *tobacco* and *alcohol* industries [*see* above], which have also tried to influence the scientific process by funding apparently independent groups. It's a conflict of interest that flies in the face of good practice.'

Coca-Cola spent €6.6 million (£4.86 million) setting up the [EHI] between 2010 and 2015. Guidance and studies it funded often recommend that the public, including children, consume sports and soft drinks of the sort sold by *Coca-Cola*. Two of the company's most senior scientists are vice-chairwomen of EHI (*see* above), whose public pages on social networks make no mention of *Coca-Cola*, although its website reveals ... that the company is a founding partner. [The] chairman of EHI's scientific advisory board is an emeritus professor of sport science at Loughborough University, which has received £817,292 from *Coca-Cola* in research funding since 2007. [He] has advised *UK Athletics* and the *Football Association*, and acted as a consultant for *Coca-Cola* and other drinks companies since the [1990s].

Through its trade organisations, *Coca-Cola* representatives met government officials and ministers more than 100 times between 2011 and 2014. The company hosts an annual parliamentary dinner. Organisations it funds often promote a message that physical activity is more important to *public health* than an 'obsession' with obesity. In 2013, [the] chairman of *UKActive*, an organisation set up to promote physical activity that lists *Coca-Cola* as a sponsor, criticised Britain for being 'fixated' by obesity at a *Coke*-organised event. [He] quoted ... a US academic whose university has received more than $3 million from *Coca-Cola*, by telling delegates: 'You can be fat and fit' [*see* Chapter 12]. *UKActive*'s board includes Baroness Grey-Thompson, [a Paralympian], Dame Carol Black [FRCP] [the Prime Minister's *adviser on health*], and Liz Lowe, *Coke GB's* director of corporate responsibility.

Coca-Cola has also given money to government advisers including ... a board member of *Food Standards Scotland.* In 2010 she co-wrote a study sponsored by the *UK Sugar Bureau*, the lobbying group for sugar manufacturers, that [reportedly] found no proven association between sugar intake and obesity [*see* above]. On her website she states separately: 'When I correlated sugar consumption with obesity levels, there didn't appear to be any relationship'. [She] said that the *UK Sugar Bureau* had *no* control over her study and that she highlighted a 'potential concern' over *sugary drinks* and obesity in the report. She said that her later comments were consistent with a recent government report and she had *not* undertaken work for *Coca-Cola* since joining *Food Standards Scotland.* She denies writing favourable reports for *Coca-Cola.* [A] professor of nutrition, food studies and public health at *New York University* said: 'In my opinion no scientist should accept funding from *Coca-Cola*. It's totally compromising.

Other government advisers who have received funding from *Coca-Cola* include [the] chairman of the state-funded scientific advisory committee on carbohydrates, who stepped down from the *Coca-Cola* advisory board [in 2012]. His university has since received a payment from EHI after he gave a talk at a hydration 'workshop'. 'I do not regard links with both *industry* and the government as being in conflict,' he said. 'Both the public and *industry* are entitled to access the *best* advice available.'

Coca-Cola Great Britain said: 'We rely on scientific research to make decisions about our products and ingredients and commission independent third parties to carry out this work'. Professor Maughan recognised 'the need for caution' over industry funding but said that much good research would not otherwise have taken place. Loughborough said its research studies were subject to a strict code of conduct.[41]

This article was accompanied by a *leading article* in the same issue of the national record:

> Rising consumption of *sugary drinks* has been a major contributor to the *obesity epidemic*. So says the website of the *Harvard School of Public Health*, citing 22 peer-reviewed articles in nearly as many leading medical journals. The *link between highly sweetened soft drinks, obesity and obesity-related disease* [my italics] is well established, not that you would know it from 'research' funded to the tune of millions of pounds by *Coca-Cola*.
>
> Systematic efforts by *Coca-Cola* to undermine solid science on the health implications of too much sugar are exposed in *The Times* ... The drinks manufacturer has invested heavily in reputable-sounding think tanks and research projects whose *Coke*-friendly findings build a case for consumption of the kinds of drinks it sells. Scientists who have accepted funding directly or indirectly from the food and drink *industry* have claimed it does not affect their findings, when research suggests otherwise.
>
> There is a broader scandal here with far-reaching implications. Obesity-related illness causes some 53,000 premature deaths, and costs the NHS about £5 billion a year. A proposal for a *sugar tax* might have eased that burden. It won the backing of ... the chief medical officer, but *was rejected this year after intensive lobbying by the UK Sugar Bureau and other pressure groups, many ... part funded by Coca-Cola* [my italics].The former chairman of *UKActive* criticised Britain at an event sponsored by *Coke* in 2013 for being 'fixated' by obesity. Public health officials are right to be fixated by obesity, and by diet as a cause of it. To argue that diet is an insignificant factor compared with physical activity, as scientists who have received funding from *Coca-Cola* often do, is to ignore a compelling mass of evidence. It is a betrayal of consumers who deserve scrupulously objective advice, and of the scientific method.

[A] nutritionist and government health adviser co-wrote a 2010 study sponsored by the *UK Sugar Bureau* from which she concluded that *'there didn't appear to be any relationship'* between sugar consumption and obesity [my italics and *see* above]. [Her] study and 17 others were subsequently reviewed by Spanish researchers who found that those sponsored by or had links to the food and drink industry were *five* times more likely than the rest to find no link between sugar and obesity.

No one is suggesting that *Coke* or its competitors be banned. Nor is there an obvious case for a draconian crackdown on commercial sponsorship of consumer-related research. There is, however, an urgent need for stricter controls. Pharmaceutical companies conduct valuable pure and applied research, and much of its value lies in the fact that the full extent of their involvement is prominently disclosed. *Coca-Cola* is opaque by comparison.

Earlier this year Loughborough University published a study [which] showed it could be more dangerous to drive when dehydrated than drunk. On the strength of this *Coca-Cola* launched a sales push for its drinks at *Shell* filling stations. As we report, it failed to note that it had previously paid [the chairman of this study] as a consultant, given more than £800,000 to his university and co-founded the think tank behind the study. *Big Tobacco* was fined billions in the US for distorting the debate on smoking. *Big Sugar* should consider itself on notice.[42]

At this point, it seemed that the British government was 'unmovable', was supporting the food industry wholeheartedly, and that a fair resolution was going to be impossible. However, the BMJ and also the *Times* heightened the campaign:

An MP and former GP has accused England's health secretary [Jeremy Hunt] of hypocrisy for refusing to publish a review of ... evidence on what measures could help to *reduce* people's consumption of sugar while claiming that he supports data sharing. In July [2015] [PHE] said that its review on controlling sugar consumption would be published at the end of the summer [to outline] the government's strategy on tackling childhood obesity. But this week the *Department of Health* said that the review and ... strategy would be published simultaneously *'in the coming months'* [my italics]. In an article in the *Daily Telegraph* on 12 October, ... the Conservative MP for Totnes and chair of the *health select committee*, called on [the] chief executive of [PHE] to use his powers to insist that the report be made public.

The agency's credibility rested on its 'freedom to set out the evidence ... without fear or favour,' she said. [The MP for Totnes] told the BMJ, '[the Health Secretary] should demonstrate his own commitment to the importance of sharing evidence in a transparent and timely manner. It cannot be right to delay ... publication of the impartial evidence review from [PHE] around measures which could reduce sugar consumption until the ink is dry on the government's strategy.' 'PHE ... must be able to exert its independence to publish even if the timing or nature of evidence is inconvenient for the government's internal debate. The problem is that, without a change of heart ... the rest of us will not know in time to make any difference.'

The Health Committee held its first evidence session on what should be included in the childhood obesity strategy on 13 October [*see* above]. Before the session [the MP for Totnes] said that committee members were 'deeply disappointed' that they had not seen the review. 'We consider that that is obstructing this inquiry,' she said.

In an update sent to the committee on 7 October [2015] the health department said that despite calls for a *tax* on sugar sweetened beverages 'we have *no* plans to introduce such a *tax*.'

[A] spokesman for the [NOF] and an adviser to *Action*

on Sugar, said, 'It is outrageous that its [PHE's evidence] should be withheld from such a vital inquiry. We can ... assume that its evidence supports the idea of a *sugary drinks tax* and that releasing the data would embarrass the British Prime Minister [David Cameron], who has already flatly, and rashly, rejected such a *tax*.' '[The Health Secretary] has already called the childhood obesity epidemic a 'great tragedy'. The greater tragedy is, however, that he appears to be conniving to hide information from fellow MPs who are desperate to overcome that *epidemic*.'[43]

A further article in the *Times* enumerated those who were either *for or against* a *sugar tax*:

For:
- Faculty of Public Health
- Public Health England
- British Medical Association
- British Heart Foundation

Against:
- David Cameron [Prime Minister]
- Food and Drink Federation
- Institute of Economic Affairs

And the newspaper's *Health Editor*, not surprisingly, continued supporting introduction of a *tax*:

A '*sugar tax*' was recommended by an official review that [the Health Secretary] has *refused to publish* [my italics], according to the government's top obesity adviser. Ministers were told that measures to limit *promotions* and 'deep, consistent' *advertising* aimed at children were even more important to tackle the problem. The *Coco Pops monkey, jumbo bags of crisps, 'bottomless' cups of fizzy drinks* and the advertising of junk food by sports stars should all be restricted or banned, the *Public Health England* paper said. The food industry must also be pressured to cut sugar levels in its products just as they did with *salt* [*see* above]. ... PHE's director of diet and obesity, told MPs yesterday. ... the health secretary, has promised that a child obesity strategy due in January [2016] will be draconian, but has faced criticism over his refusal to publish PHE's analysis of the evidence for the measures. [PHE's director of diet and obesity] revealed that the review concluded that 'universally all the evidence shows that *tax* does decrease purchases' as she outlined its contents to the Commons health select committee. 'PHE does see there is a role for a fiscal approach in reducing sugary drink consumption. The higher the *tax* increase the greater the effect,' she said, pointing out that in Mexico a *fizzy drinks tax* led to a 6 per cent fall in sales, with the biggest impact on the poorest. 'The point of the *tax* is to nudge people away from purchasing these things … that are more consistent with a healthy balanced diet,' she said.

[The PHE's director of diet and obesity] stressed that *tax* was only the fourth most effective way to fight obesity. 'We think there could be bigger impacts from getting a handle on *promotions*, and of getting a handle on the deep, consistent *advertising* our children are exposed to on unhealthy foods,' she said. About 40% of food is discounted and such deals are heavily weighted towards sweet and fatty products, … research found. She said that such promotions did not cut costs for consumers but simply 'lead to us buying more food'. She added: 'PHE are advising that promotions need to be restricted and rebalanced if we want to reduce sugar consumption.' Rules that limit *junk food* advertising on children's TV 'are not deep enough,' [she] argued. She said that it was wrong that rules prevented only branded cartoon characters from being deployed to *advertise* junk to kids 'so *Dumbo* can't be (deployed) but the *Coco Pops* money can be. Yet the evidence is that things like those *Coco Pops monkeys* do engage children and affect food choice.' She said that sponsorship of sports events by *fizzy drinks* and the use of 'sports heroes' to sell unhealthy food should be targeted. *'I'm very worried that we're beginning to see practices that we commonly see in the [USA] coming into the UK* [my italics]. For example, we're seeing bottomless cups in some restaurants,' she said. 'Single bags of crisps are substantially larger than they were 15 years ago. I don't think many of us need those crisps at the bottom of the packet.'

One child in five is obese by the time they leave primary school and [the Health Secretary] has made fighting childhood obesity a priority. [He] warned that focusing on primary school children alone would not solve the problem.[44]

The British government seemed therefore now to be of the persuasion that *under no circumstance would it implement a 'sugar tax'*!

The health minister (Jeremy Hunt) on behalf of the government however, continued with suppression of the PHE report, believing that *'refined-sugar'* reduction was only one of several ways of reducing obesity. However, the London Mayor (Boris Johnson), a prominent Conservative politician (by then also an MP), opposed the government's position,[45] and this was followed by yet another *Times* (first) leading article:

In July [2015] the health secretary, was handed a report by [PHE] into how best to reduce the nation's sugar intake. This is an issue of grave concern: excess sugar consumption is an important factor in obesity. Obesity-related illness is linked to 53,000 premature deaths each year and costs the NHS more than £5 billion annually to treat. [The London Mayor's] assertion that he is 'thinking seriously' about a *sugar tax* to help tackle the issue may be political mischief-making. However, it is also a welcome contribution to the debate and [PHE]'s report is timely. It is therefore dismaying that [the Health Secretary – Hunt] has thus far neglected to publish it. He should do so without further delay.

The impact of obesity is particularly troubling on the young. By the time they leave primary school, one in five children is obese. [The Health Secretary] has promised to publish the PHE's report in January [2016], alongside a national strategy for dealing with childhood obesity [*see* below]. There is no reason to link the two. In the meantime

... the director of diet and obesity at PHE has provided [a] welcome insight. Having spent a year analysing 23 different sugar-reduction policies in use worldwide, this week she told the House of Commons select committee on health that the evidence shows that *taxing sugar* reduces consumption. The higher the *tax*, the bigger the decrease. This will be uncomfortable news for the government, which recently ruled out imposing a *sugar tax*. Citing an unwillingness to raise the cost of living, its decision was welcomed by the *Food and Drink Federation*. The reluctance to introduce a *tax* that runs the risk of being regressive is understandable. The *Faculty of Public Health*, [PHE], the *British Medical Association* and the *British Heart Foundation* all support a *sugar tax*. *As an exasperated Jamie Oliver [see above and below] asked the Commons health committee this week: 'Who is running the country? The businesses who are profiting from ill health, or us?'* [my italics].

Mexico could provide one template. It has implemented a *tax* on *fizzy drinks* containing sugar and seen a 6% decline in sales. There is evidence that obesity is linked to a high intake of sugar-sweetened drinks. A single can of *fizzy drink* can contain up to *14* teaspoons of sugar, double the daily recommended intake for adults. Government advice is that no more than 5% of our daily calories should come from sugar, yet for many of us that figure is closer to 10%. *Many tinned soups, salad dressings and low-fat foods contain unexpected 'hidden' amounts of sugar* [my italics]. In her evidence to MPs, [the PHE's director of diet and obesity] made an interesting comparison with the successful attempts over the past decade to encourage the food industry to cut levels of *salt* [see above]. This resulted in a 15% reduction in *salt* intake and an estimated reduction in ... content of supermarket foods of between 20% and 40%. There is no reason why sugar cannot undergo a similar trajectory.

Reducing our consumption of sugar is a matter of personal choice as much as government edict. Consumers must become better informed on the dangers of excessive consumption and manufacturers could be more transparent about sugar content. The government and retailers must consider ways of encouraging us to make better choices, as they did with plastic bags. Tighter regulation of advertising and promotions is one such tool, particularly with regards to those aimed at children. It is possible that the use of *sports stars* to promote *junk food* should be restricted or banned, and supermarkets should refrain from stocking checkouts with sweets at a child's eye level. This is a complex issue, however. [PHE]'s report may contain some of the answers. *It deserves a wider readership than the secretary of state for health* [my italics].[46]

In late October 2015, a solution to this highly contentious issue which was still facing the British government seemed to divide itself into:

- Whether to allow an *individual* choice (*ie,* whether or *not* to make ingestion of *'refined-sugar'* a personal issue) – as was the case in the *tobacco* debate, or
- Would a *'sugar-tax'* introduce 'nanny-state' mentality, as was so prevalent during the 'Blair/Brown' era of the previous *Labour* government.

Would the British government therefore, impose a 'sugar-tax' as had been the case with tobacco?
The decision at this point lay squarely on the *Conservative* Government. Which way would it elect to jump?

Summary of the tax situation in late 2015

As early as mid-2014, the reader of the *Sunday Times* had been informed of a *'leaked report'*, commissioned by the *Department of Health*, calling for a *tax* on *sugary drinks* and *'foods with a high sugar content'*. This *draft* report suggested that a '20% *tax* on sugar-sweetened drinks … could reduce consumption and prevalence of obesity in adults by 1.3% (*see* above). However the *Department of Health* had already indicated that the government '… had *no* plans to introduce a *sugar tax'*. Meanwhile, the *Tesco* chief had 'privately "lobbied" government to introduce a law to tackle obesity'. *Tesco* (he claimed) was 'exploring ways' to support the government's ... campaign to *reduce calories*' (my italics). However, the *Department of Health* had already indicated that it would 'help people to make healthier choices' *before* deciding that a *sugar tax* was really necessary.

Effects of the 'obesity epidemic' on inability to finance the NHS was becoming of huge concern. So many were affected by obesity, or perhaps more specifically its complications, that a forecast confidently predicted that during the following two decades, more hospitals would be necessary, at a cost of 'billions of pounds'. As an example, NHS staff who were overweight were being compulsorily put on diets, in order that they 'practise what [they] preach' (*see* Chapter 13). Not only doctors, but nurses, porters, and managers would be offered a twelve-week *Slimming World* course as part of a plan to advise overweight individuals on 'dieting, cookery lessons and [even] dance on the NHS'. Meanwhile, many diets sold to the public were described by 'experts' as mere 'nutribabble'; not only did they lack 'long-term' implications but were frequently 'drowned out' by *industry* marketing' to simply raise money.

The UK's shadow health secretary, and at that time a *potential* leader of the Labour party (Jeremy Corbyn), had been reported on 20 June 2014 as promising to 'impose limits' on the quantity of '*refined-sugar*' in breakfast cereals, *if elected*, but this was *not* apparently mentioned in the Labour party's *public health* manifesto!

The position in late October 2015 had become politically polarised: *should, or should not a tax be imposed on 'sugary' food and drink?* It should be recalled that *all* manufactured foods contain *some* sugar. Thus, by imposing a *sugar tax* it is the *poor* and *not* the *rich* who were in danger of suffering the greatest penalty! Jamie Oliver – the high profile chef – had already decided (with limited success) to impose a 10p *tax* on *all* sugary drinks sold in his restaurants. This strategy was similarly employed by 'hospitals, restaurants and councils'. He also suggested a 7p sugar-tax nationally, which would of course require *legislation*. On the other hand, by no means everyone agreed that a *tax* would lead to weight reduction, for with *tobacco* it was *education* and *not* financial factors which [eventually] led to the steep reduction; if this had been entirely dependent on *taxation* that would have had to be extremely high! This conclusion was borne out by imposition of a *tobacco*-tax in Mexico, and a *saturated fat-tax* in Denmark. The fiscal brunt of a *taxation policy* would therefore probably have greatest impact on poorer classes – who in any case would *continue* to purchase 'sugary food(s)'.

Progress of the saga in 2016

By the latter part of 2015, the question of a 'sugar tax' had thus come to the fore in the British media and was a high profile topic. The 'quality' newspapers were inundated with contributions, and it is *no* exaggeration to conclude that the vast majority favoured a *tax*; but how much should it be? Both the *sugar industry* and government remained at loggerheads with the 'common man'. In early January 2016, the *Times* published the following as its *first* leading article:

> Even in the upper echelons of government few have the power to save thousands of lives by championing one policy over another. ... the health secretary could save tens of thousands of lives and tens of billions of pounds for the taxpayer by facing up to the gravity of Britain's *obesity epidemic*. This entails cajoling consumers to eat better while heaping pressure on food manufacturers to cut levels of harmful ingredients. It requires tough *legislative* action, too.
>
> Excessive sugar consumption is closely linked to obesity, which ... the NHS chief has called '*the new smoking*'. Obesity is a prime cause of *type-2-diabetes*, which afflicts nearly four million adults – an increase of 70 per cent in a decade – and directly or indirectly costs the [NHS] more than £10 billion a year. It is time for [the Health Secretary] to accept the advice of two thirds of GPs and his most senior *public health* officials and insist on a *tax* on sugar.
>
> The proportion of Britons who are obese or overweight may be a symptom of prosperity. It is also a national scandal affecting a quarter of young children, a third of 11–15-year-olds and two thirds of adults. Inadequate *exercise* is a factor, but poor diet is the main culprit. The levels of physical

activity needed to rid our collective waistline of its excess pounds would be 'literally Olympic' [*see* Chapter 12], the head of *Diabetes UK* tells *The Times* ... We are what we eat. Too much fat contributes to obesity, but cutting back on sugar is the single most efficient strategy for losing weight and limiting the risk of diabetes and its complications. These complications include heart disease, kidney failure, blindness, loss of hearing and amputations [*see* Chapter 11]. Obesity more broadly is [also] closely correlated with a high risk of cancer, liver disease and depression. Diabetes and diabetes-related illnesses alone consume a tenth of the NHS budget and cause 24,000 premature deaths a year.

This is a *public health* disaster that has expanded incrementally, but an incremental response will not suffice. Last year [the British Prime Minister – David Cameron] rejected the idea of a *sugar tax* when it was proposed by [PHE] as one of *eight* courses of action that would cut the nation's intake. PHE's other proposals include a ban on *advertising* high-sugar food to children and strict limits on two-for-one offers of *confectionary* [sic] and *fizzy drinks*. Such ideas are likely to be included in the government's forthcoming *child obesity strategy* [my italics]. As things stand, a *sugar tax* is not.

[The Prime Minister] is thought to oppose a *tax* because he fears being seen to penalise poorer households that consume large quantities of high-sugar foods. He should not take fright so easily. If a *sugar tax* hits the poor hardest, they will see its benefits most clearly too. It is, in any case, the height of condescension to assume that the less well-off are also less able to improve their diets in response to good advice. ... the former chief medical officer [Sir Liam Donaldson has] argued strongly for a *tax* .... [Cameron] has been coy in public but is thought privately to favour one. It is reasonable to worry that an unduly complicated *tax* would be too expensive to enforce, but a 10% *tax* on *high-sugar fizzy drinks* would be a simple and practical starting point.

It is time for a *sugar tax* because nothing else is working. As academics and the PHE's chief nutritionist told parliament last year [2015] public education and voluntary agreements with the food industry all have a role but so far have failed to cut sugar consumption.

Smoking in cinemas and restaurants used to be accepted with barely a murmur. Now it is hard to imagine. As [the Health Secretary – Hunt] fine-tunes his *child obesity strategy*, he should consider whether he wants to be remembered as a health secretary shackled by inertia or one who followed the dictates of reason and insisted on reform.[47]

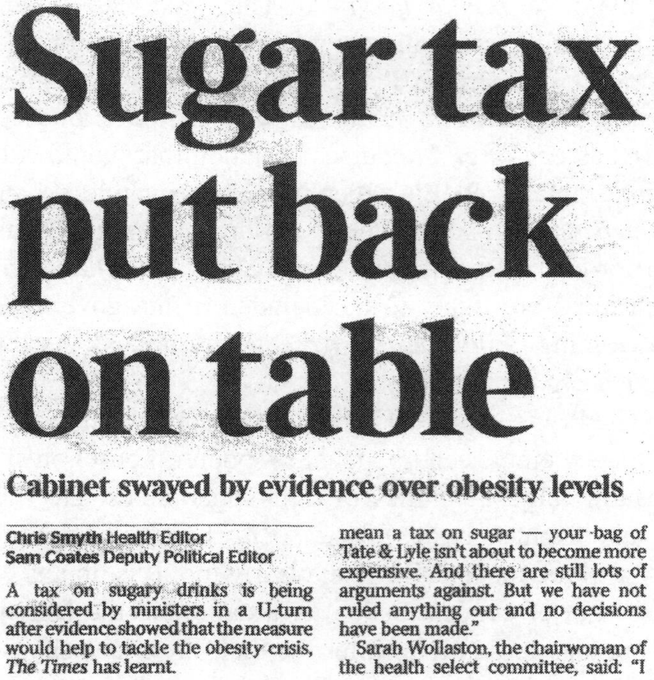

Sugar tax put back on table

Cabinet swayed by evidence over obesity levels

Chris Smyth Health Editor
Sam Coates Deputy Political Editor

A tax on sugary drinks is being considered by ministers in a U-turn after evidence showed that the measure would help to tackle the obesity crisis, *The Times* has learnt.

mean a tax on sugar — your bag of Tate & Lyle isn't about to become more expensive. And there are still lots of arguments against. But we have not ruled anything out and no decisions have been made."

Sarah Wollaston, the chairwoman of the health select committee, said: "I

Fig 16.2: Headline in the London *Times* newspaper: a *sugar-tax* is not far off! (*Times, Lond*; 2016 January 7: 1, 10.)

208

The possibility of a 20% *'sugar tax'* apparently fuelled an 'internal battle' at 10 Downing Street (the Head of WHO had also called for introduction of a *sugar tax*), so that 'a failure to act would have major medical, social and economic consequences', was their considered opinion.[48] Although the Prime Minister had ruled out a *tax* the previous year (2015), in January 2016 'taxes were [apparently] back on the table'; this followed the Mexican evidence that a 10% *tax* had led to a 12% fall in sugar sales.[49] A *Times* main banner headline in early 2016 read: **Sugar tax put back on table: cabinet swayed by evidence over obesity levels**. It seemed therefore to most *Times* readers that it was merely a matter of time before government introduced a *tax on sugar* (*see* fig 16.2).[50]

In February 2016, publicity attempts to impose a 20% *sugar-tax* were promoted by high profile campaigns:

- Jamie Oliver (*see* above) was interviewed on the BBC's 'Andrew Marr programme' on 7 February 2016 reiterating his assertion that excessive sugar – especially in childhood – was detrimental to health. He furthermore steadfastly supported a *'sugar tax'* and had by then become a leading figure in the campaign, and
- Jeremy Hunt (British Health Secretary) was interviewed on the same programme – his main argument emanating from the standpoint of a significant financial saving for the *NHS*, which was currently in a *critical* state.

The proposed *tax* was also strongly supported by a 'British Olympic Star' – James Cracknell.[51]

Such a *tax* had apparently been accepted in principle by supermarkets and 'fast food outlets', but the ultimate decision had obviously to be taken by *HM Government*. Surprisingly, despite this long fought campaign against *'refined-sugar'*, sales had actually *increased*.

- *Coca-Cola* appeared to be making progress in its attempts to win back health-conscious consumers who were spurning its sugary drinks,
- The *Coca-Cola* Company had reported a 6% *increase* in world-wide sales of non-carbonated drinks such as tea, bottled water

and ready-to-drink coffee in the fourth quarter of 2015,

- [*Coca Cola*] also reported progress in its '*fizzy drinks*', with a quarterly volume growth of 2% worldwide. Increased sales of *Sprite* and *Coca-Cola Zero* were only partially offset by declines in *Diet Coke* and *Coca-Cola Light,*
- The company [had] reported a better-than-expected profit of $1.24 billion for the quarter, a rise from $700 million a year earlier, helped by aggressive cost-cutting and higher pricing.
- ... *Coca-Cola*'s chief executive indicated that its North American division [had] the previous year [2015] delivered its strongest annual performance in three years, and
- *Coca-Cola's* shares were up half of one per cent at $42.88 ....[52]

In mid-February 2016, the following *almost unbelievable* report appeared in the *Times* newspaper:

The government has *ruled out* proposals for a *sugar tax* to help ... tackle Britain's obesity crisis, it was reported last night. [The British Prime Minister – David Cameron] has been considering a levy of up to 20% as *part* of his anti-obesity strategy but claims surfaced that *he is* set to give the food industry *another chance to develop healthier products of its own accord* [my italics]. The threat of the *tax* would be retained to encourage producers to make swift changes. No 10 [Downing Street] last night said that no final decision had been taken but it is understood that there was an internal discussion in Downing Street over whether or not to deliver a verdict *before* the [*European Union* referendum in June 2016 – *see* below]. One senior figure said: 'It is a finely balanced decision'. Some ministers believe that the *food industry* is trying to pressure the government into making a snap decision. [The Prime Minister] is expected to unveil the *obesity strategy* towards the end of the month. Drinks companies will be expected to reformulate their products to reduce sugar content, with the prospect of a future *tax* if they fail to meet targets, according to the *Financial Times.*

Kellogg's and *Coca-Cola* were among brands [which] last month promised to cut the sugar content of their products. The makers of *Lucozade* and *Ribena* are aiming to cut sugar by 10% by 2018. It has been estimated that a 20% sugar *tax* could raise up to ... £1 billion a year.[53]

The 2016 Budget

To most people's surprise and delight, taking into account previous jittering, on 16 March (2016) (*Budget Day*) a *tax* on 'sugary food' was at last announced by the *Chancellor of the Exchequer* (George Osborne) as one component of his 'cuts'. Whether the decision had been taken by the Chancellor or the Prime Minister remains unclear. The following day the London *Times* newspaper launched its report with the main front page headline in large, bold typeface – **Osborne sugars the pill** (*see* fig 16.3).[54]

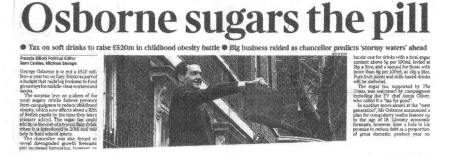

Fig 16.3: *Times* post-2016 Budget headline. *Osborne was Chancellor of the Exchequer.* (*Times, Lond* 2016; March 17: 1, 2.)

Not before time, therefore, the British government had pushed aside the *sugar industry* which had at last 'lost out'. The *sugar tax*, it was said, could add 8p to the cost of a 'fizzy drink' – when introduced in April 2018. Drinks with a *total* sugar content above 5g 100m l⁻¹ would be taxed at 18p l⁻¹, and others with >8 mg 100 ml l⁻¹ at 24p l⁻¹. It was estimated that a *tax* on soft drinks would raise £520 million for the national economy. The drinks *industry* was, not surprisingly, however in uproar! Meanwhile an accompanying columnist welcomed the decision and a leading article entitled 'Unsweetened Medicine' maintained that '[Osborne's] *eighth* budget will be remembered firstly for its *sugar tax*'.

In a 'market report' in the same newspaper, introduction of the sugar levy had apparently '... sent shares in the sector lower ...'; several examples being given. However, it was anticipated that 'the *tax* would be passed on to consumers, and therefore the impact would ultimately depend on consumer preference and reaction'. Reactions from manufacturers were outlined in an accompanying article: '... the industry reacted furiously hinting that companies could [perhaps] abandon *voluntary* efforts to make products healthier. Meanwhile, 'Experts said that the introduction of a *sugar tax* on soft drinks raised the prospect of *taxes* on other products such as sweets and chocolate bars'. A spokesman for the *Food and Drink Federation*, while dismissing its effect on obesity, considered the *tax* was merely a 'piece of political theatre'.[55]

The following day however, a correspondent from NOF, *not* entirely happy with this outcome, maintained that a 'swifter and more dramatic outcome' would have resulted by 'slapping tough levies on [manufacturers] that lace their products with ['*refined-sugar*'] for the 'higher the *tax*, the greater [would be] the fall in consumption'.[56]

Conclusions as Cameron 'stepped down' as Prime Minister
There is therefore an overwhelming acknowledgement that '*refined-sugar*' had had a large part to play in the *obesity epidemic,* and that earlier introduction of a 20% 'sugar *tax*' would have done much to solve this problem sooner. One is left with the unpalatable conclusion that the (*Conservative*) government was far more interested in supporting the *food industry*, and its shareholders, than the health of the future citizens of Britain. Thus, politicians are certainly *not* to be trusted on health matters.

A new Prime Minister (and government): plans for dealing with the obesity epidemic overruled and in disarray!
On 23 June 2016 the British *European Union* (EU) referendum had been held, and was unexpectedly won by those wishing to exit. Prime Minister Cameron (and his government) resigned, and the childless Theresa May (1956–present) became the unelected Prime Minister, who formed the new administration. Philip Hammond (1955–present) became *Chancellor of the Exchequer*.

In several ways, 2016 had perhaps proved to be the most important year in the British 'fight over the *obesity pandemic'*. There had been repeated calls for something to be done by the British government: should a *tax* be imposed on all 'sugary' food and drinks? Arguments *for* and *against* taxation by influential figures had been vociferous. Eventually, a *tax* had been imposed by the *Chancellor of the Exchequer* (Osborne) in his annual budget; this was welcomed by all of those supportive of the war *against* obesity, as well as supporters of the NHS on which obesity and its complications (especially *type-2-diabetes*) was costing so much! Furthermore, the *elected* British Prime Minister – Cameron – had worked out his future strategy (involving *advertising* and *promotion* of sweet food and drink) to minimise obesity (especially that affecting children) in England.

In late 2016, the momentum however immediately changed. In the London *Times* newspaper, the principal headline on August 18 was: **May rips up plans for junk-food crackdown** (*see* Prologue). The article began:

> Tough measures to tackle obesity have been axed after Theresa May overruled the health secretary and insisted that the *economy* must take priority. Restrictions on advertising and promotional deals on *junk food* have been removed from a plan published today. This is despite [PHE's] insistence that such steps would be the most effective way to prevent children getting fat.
>
> "It's been castrated," one Whitehall source said. Experts and campaigners also reacted with outrage at the move. A push by Jeremy Hunt, the health secretary, for "draconian" action was rejected by No 10. It is understood that Downing Street does not want to burden the *food industry* as the economy falters. Lobbyists argue that reduced revenues could lead to job losses. ...
>
> Measures over advertising and promotions appear nowhere in the plan, which puts an emphasis on encouraging children to do more *exercise.*

This decision was one of the first to abolish 'one by one' those policies inherited from her predecessor! Also, in October (2016) London's *Sunday Times* carried the headline: *'May takes bite out of child obesity fight'* (*see* fig 16.4).[57] Precisely why she had taken this stance is difficult to comprehend; May is herself a *diabetes* victim (albeit a type-1 rather than type-2 sufferer) and the NHS was seriously overburdened financially – largely as a result of the obesity epidemic accompanied by its major complication, type-2-diabetes.[58] Therefore May's administration, Britain's *new* governing body, had declared a total lack of interest in the health of the country's future generation!

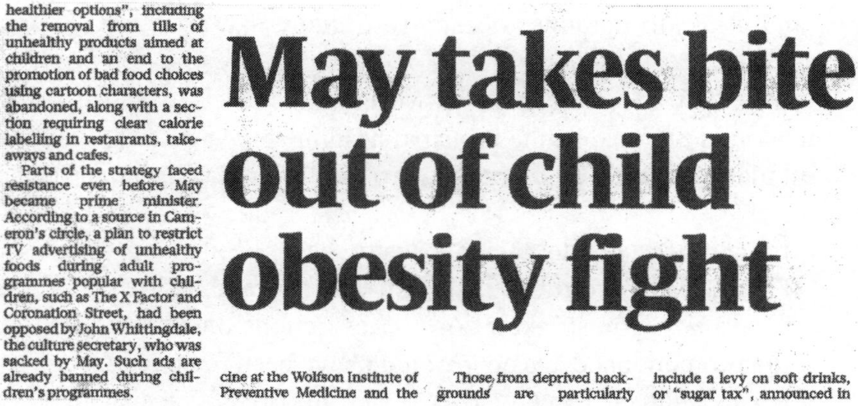

healthier options", including the removal from tills of unhealthy products aimed at children and an end to the promotion of bad food choices using cartoon characters, was abandoned, along with a section requiring clear calorie labelling in restaurants, takeaways and cafes.

Parts of the strategy faced resistance even before May became prime minister. According to a source in Cameron's circle, a plan to restrict TV advertising of unhealthy foods during adult programmes popular with children, such as The X Factor and Coronation Street, had been opposed by John Whittingdale, the culture secretary, who was sacked by May. Such ads are already banned during children's programmes.

May takes bite out of child obesity fight

cine at the Wolfson Institute of Preventive Medicine and the

Those from deprived backgrounds are particularly

include a levy on soft drinks, or "sugar tax", announced in

Fig 16.4: Newspaper headline shortly after appointment of the incoming prime minister, May (*Sunday Times*, *Lond* 2016; October 30: 12.)

Calls for a *tax* on sugary food and 'fizzy drinks' had begun several years in the past and were certainly in 'full swing' by 2015. The obesity epidemic was in one way or another threatening the demise of Britain's NHS, and numerous individuals and organisations had been lobbying for a *'sugar tax'*. A distinct lack of interest from the British government had thus come as a bitter disappointment.[59] But the new Prime Minister clearly had other priorities in mind and accumulated evidence suggests that the *obesity epidemic* was well down this list! Although more drastic action on sugar still seems likely, who can tell what will ensue while May holds the exalted office of Prime Minister!

2017 and the 2017 budget

In March 2017 Hammond delivered the annual ('botched' or 'U-turn') Budget – the last *Spring* Budget! One section relating to the *sugar tax* was reported the following day (March 17) in London's *Times* newspaper:

> The *sugar tax* [due in April 2018] will raise £135 million a year less than expected because *fizzy drinks* manufacturers are scrambling to make their products healthier, the chancellor said yesterday. He said the levy would be set at 18p a litre on drinks with more than 5g of sugar per 100 ml, such as *Fanta* and *Sprite,* and 24p for those with more than 8g per 100 ml, such as *Coca-Cola.* 'Unusually for a chancellor, I am delighted to announce a reduction in the expected yield of a *tax*,' he said. 'Producers are already reformulating sugar out of their drinks, which means a lower revenue forecast' ...
>
> The Treasury now estimates it will raise £385 million in the year after it is introduced in April 2018; down from the £520 million originally envisioned. The money is earmarked for school sports and Mr Hammond promised to top up funding so that children's programmes did not lose out from the lower revenue ...
>
> Over a quarter of a teenager's daily added sugar intake comes from soft drinks, and they have no nutritional benefit at all. A study last year found that the *tax* could prevent one in ten cases of child obesity in Britain.

The inevitable consequence came in March 2017 when 'food giants' decided to ignore deliberations of parliament and impose their own strategy to deal with the situation. They obviously had to accept the *sugar tax* (agreed in 2016) but other measures in Cameron's plan (*ie,* to reduce sugar in drinks by one fifth by 2020) were 'watered down', *eg,* his tough imposition of a strict timetable of '*refined-sugar*' restriction within a specified period were abandoned while the *food industry*'s own arbitrary dates were substituted.

Thus May's rejection of Cameron's tough 'blue-print' in 2016 again played directly into the hands of the *food industry* and overruled common-sense aims of Britain's *public health* establishment. A spokesman for the industry also suggested that dietary items other than '*refined-sugar*' remained under suspicion regarding the *aetiology* of obesity (and also presumably the rising incidence of childhood caries).[60] Britain was thus left with a *sugar tax* (to be introduced in 2018) but with none of Cameron's other intentions – including limitation of *advertising* and *promotional* campaigns!

There were immediate reactions to this soft and watered-down response (only 13 instead of 37 pages) by the administration led by May. The '*sugar tax*' was of course supported by the new government, but *advertising* and *promotion* had been removed from the report on prevention of childhood obesity. Reliance was therefore placed on a 'dishonest' *sugar industry* for *voluntary* reduction of sugar content; however, no *timescale* had been laid down, and the *soft drinks* industry was thus delighted. The *new* Prime Minister had put *economy* ahead of children's health (and therefore the future population of Britain).

The *food industry* has a long history of lobbying the government of the day; towards the end of his time as Prime Minister, Cameron 'caved in' and introduced a *sugar tax*. May began her period as Prime Minister by making the disastrous decision of disregarding the next generation, and disallowed sugar *advertising* and *promotion* to proceed, and instead wholeheartedly backed the country's *economy*. She has in effect dismantled Government regulation of the *sugar industry* and relied on *voluntary* strategies instead of imposing strict control. This is comparable to voluntary regulation of *salt*-content of foodstuffs (*see* above) – which was a totally different matter. May also neglected the fact that *type-2-diabetes* which at the time was costing the NHS (and therefore the country's *economy*) a vast financial sum which had the potential to sink the NHS!

In the debates upon dietary factors responsible for the *obesity epidemic*, it is important to emphasise that *education* and *not* taxation is in any case ultimately essential for a solution. And furthermore, *most* 2017 foodstuffs do contain *some* '*refined-sugar*'. Much discussion has involved aspects of physical fitness: are we also *drinking* (alcohol) and *smoking* too much, and also ingesting an excessive quantity of *salt*, each of which is known to be potentially harmful, and to impose (directly or indirectly) financial strains upon an overstretched NHS. So is there anything to be learned from efforts to reduce consumption of these undesirable items? All are in fact components of *public health* delivery, about which the present government seems to have little interest.

In late March 2017 (*ie,* some *nine* months after May replaced Cameron's strategy with a plan based on 'goodwill' from the *sugar industry* and without any compulsion whatsoever), PHE – a government advisory body on health matters – issued *voluntary* guidelines to the *sugar industry* to reduce '*refined-sugar*' content in *all* food products (highlighting breakfast cereals and chocolate bars) by 20% in *three* years (*ie,* by March 2020). If not satisfactorily implemented, it added, *legislation* will inevitably follow! Presumably by March 2017, the *industry* had become convinced that '*refined-sugar*' had a part to play in the obesity pandemic. PHE was apparently of the dubious persuasion that in a comparison with *salt* restriction (*see* above), *gradual* reduction in sugar would *not* be noticed by the consumer![61]

In *summary*, the British government – under the stewardship of two prime ministers – reluctantly instituted *three* measures to exert influence over the obesity *crisis*:

1   improved *education* – which has *not* proved particularly successful so far,

2   levy on *soft drinks* (the '*sugar tax*') to be introduced in
April 2018, and

3   *requests* to the food industry to *voluntarily* reduce
'*refined-sugar*' content of food by 20% by 2020. In the
event of this target *not* being achieved, more draconian action, such as more *legislation*, will possibly be
imposed.[62]

The parallel with *salt* restriction is repeatedly quoted, but the two are dissimilar. To throw this matter back to the 'goodwill' of the *industry* seems rash, but government's intention will hopefully be revealed by 2020 – hopefully by a *new* Prime Minister!

References and notes

1   J R Ashton, C Askew, N Modi, J Wass. Obesity strategy 'is long overdue'. *Times, Lond* 2016; March 2: 26.

2   C Smyth. Halve sugar intake for a healthier life. *Ibid* 2014; March 6: 7; M Syed. I won't be giving up sugar – and that's my responsibility. *Ibid* 2014; May 1: 28; C Smyth. Five a day might not be enough to keep doctor away. *Ibid* 2014; April 1: 16; R Bennett. Lose more weight with a tailored diet. *Ibid* 2014; June 2: 15; R Bennett. Sugar fears cause drop in fizzy pop sales. *Ibid* 2014; July 30: 19; H Devlin. Dieting may make you healthier, not happier. *Ibid* 2014; August 7: 15; K Lay. Fruit juices are too sugary to be included in five-a-day. *Ibid* 2014; November 11: 7; K Lay. Britons lose zest for juices high in sugar. *Ibid* 2014; December 10: 21; C Smyth. Dump the lumps with sugar swaps, wage health chiefs. *Ibid* [2014]; January 5: 4; D Hipwell. Sugar dip sweetens world food prices *Ibid* 2014; April 3: 50.

3   K Mansey, J Ungoed-Thomas. Leaked report calls for tax onslaught on sugary drinks. *Sunday Times, Lond* 2014; June 15: 7.

4   A Clark. Life is sweet despite huge fall in profits from sugar. *Times, Lond* 2014; November 5: 41.

5   C Smyth. Wine and beer labels should show calories. *Ibid* 2014; October 31: 28.

6   H Sage. Winemakers see red over calorie counts. *Ibid* 2015; April 23: 35.

7   Anonymous. The Nation's Health: Better to prevent smoking, heavy drinking and obesity than withdraw treatment. *Ibid* 2015; January 1: 26; C Smyth. It's time we took some sensible risks with our health. *Ibid* 2016; January 8: 28.

8   C Smyth. Food industry's failure to reduce salt is costing thousands of lives. *Ibid* 2015; April 29: 6; A Barnett. Is your health food too salty to be good for you? *Times 2, Lond* 2015; April 30: 5; J Lazarus, S Bath, E Combet, J Hickey. Salt dangers. *Times, Lond* 2015; May 5: 28; J Boswell. 'Misleading' child meals list salt limits. *Sunday Times, Lond* 2016; February 21: 13; G A McGregor, F J He, S Pombo-Rodrigues. How the salt reduction strategy was derailed. *Br med J* 350; 20–2.

9   S Harris. *What have plants ever done for us? Western civilisation in fifty plants.* Oxford: Bodleian Library 2015: 122–5; A M Shane. The

new world of tobacco. *History Today* 2017; 67(4): 41–7.

10 C Smyth, S Coates. Ration healthcare for smokers, alcoholics and obese, say voters 2015, *Times, Lond* January 1: 13. M Savage. Sweet-makers warn of plain packet fears. *Ibid* 2015: July 25: 6.

11 S Jebb. Tobacco can show us the way to tackle our obesity disaster. *Ibid* 2015; March 16: 26; D Walsh. Tobacco giant 'paid bribes' to protect sales in Africa. *Ibid* 2015; December 1: 9; K Lay, A Frean. Doctors accuse food companies of acting like Big Tobacco. *Ibid* 2015; April 23: 19.

12 P Sever. Our obesity epidemic and the food industry. *Ibid* 2014; January 11: 25.

13 R Bennett. 'Drinkorexics' lose weight by replacing food with alcohol. *Ibid* 2015; February 10: 21; G Matten, A Goggins. Wine, chocolate, capers: 20 foods that can make you slimmer. *Times 2, Lond* 2016; January 4: 4–5; A Sage. Wine-makers see red; J Naish. Is your wine habit really a health risk? 20 things you should know before sipping … *Ibid* 2014; August 12: 6–7; C Smyth. Alcohol has no health benefits after all. *Times, Lond* 2015; February 11: 6; C Smyth. Single drink is one too many, warn health chiefs. *Ibid* 2016; January 8: 1, 4; R Musgrave. Alcohol limits. *Ibid* 2016; January 11: 26; N P Hudd. Determining the risks of drinking alcohol. *Ibid* 2016; January 9: 24; I Knight. You polish your halo. I'll buff my wine glass and pour. *Sunday Times, Lond* 2016; January 10: 27; Anonymous. New alcohol warning. *Times. Lond* 2016; January 10: 33; C Smyth. Healthier eating saves middle-class drinkers. *Ibid* 2016; February 18: 5.

14 C Smyth. Make snacking shameful again, says obesity chief. *Ibid* 2015; March 16: 10.

15 J Ungoed-Thomas, J Stoneman. Pupils taught cola is part of a healthy diet. *Sunday Times, Lond* 2015; May 24: 13; R Ballam. British Nutrition Foundation explains what goes on the 'eatwell' plate. *Ibid* 2015; May 31: 26.

16 A Mostrous. Fizzy drinks giant pays millions to diet experts: scandal as scientists deny sugar link with obesity *Times, Lond* 2015; October 9: 1,9.

17 J Gornall. Sugar: Spinning a web of influence: public health scientists are involved with firms blamed for the obesity crisis. *Br med J* 2015;

350 (February 14): 15–17.

18 J Yudkin. *Pure, white and deadly: how sugar is killing us and what we can do to stop it*. London: Penguin Books 1986: 166–88.

19 C Smyth. Sugar is the new tobacco, say doctors. *Times, Lond* 2014; January 9: 7.

20 C Smyth. Lansley ridicules claims that sugar is the new tobacco. *Ibid* 2014; January 10: 5; F Gibb. Appeal judges order release of Lansley's diaries. *Ibid* 2017; May 25: 12.

21 J Turner. We are too sweet on sugar to give it up easily. *Ibid* 2014; January 11: 23.

22 Op cit. *See* note 12 above.

23 Anonymous. Tesco's health kick. *Times, Lond* 2015; January 7: 33.

24 J Preston. Obesity? We have only ourselves to blame. *Ibid* 2015; January 15: 25.

25 S Griffiths, T Shipman. Hospitals join Jamie with 7p tax on sugar. *Sunday Times, Lond* 2015; October 25: 10; T Whipple. Hospitals already impose a sugar tax, says Oliver. *Times, Lond* 2015; October 26: 21; S Griffiths. Jamie fears PM's war on sugar may dissolve. *Sunday Times, Lond* 2016; February 7: 5; J Oliver. The PM must stand up to Big Food and save our kids from sugar. *Times, Lond* 2016; February 7: 19; M Savage. Jamie Oliver: I will fight Tories if they fail on obesity. *Ibid* 2016; February 8: 6.

26 J Gaskin. Obesity? We have only ourselves to blame. *Ibid 2015*; January 15: 25.

27 B Kingston. *Ibid*.

28 G Jones. Sugar. *Ibid* 2014; January 14: 27.

29 J Ungoed-Thomas, K Mansey. Sugar advisors have their cake and eat it. *Sunday Times, Lond* 2014; January 19: 12.

30 Op cit. *See* note 18 above.

31 Op cit. *See* note 4 above.

32 Anonymous. Sugary challenge. *New Scientist* 2014; January 18: 4

33 G Iacobucci. Incentivise GPs to tackle obesity, doctors urge UK government. *Br med J* 2014; 348 (January 18): 3.

34 D Cohen. Sports drinks adverts are banned for false claims. *Times, Lond*; 348 (January 18): 5.

35 Op cit. *See* note 32 above.

36 J Reynolds. Sugary foods face being taxed, minister warns. *Times, Lond* 2015; May 22: 23.

37 H Devlin. Tax to take fizz out of sugary drinks and help obese. *Ibid* 2013; November 1:13.

38 Anonymous. Sugar is addictive, warns top doctor. *Ibid* 2014; March 5: 4.

39 Anonymous. Fat tax boosted healthier eating. *Ibid* 2015; May 9: 33.

40 Op cit. *See* note 3 above.

41 A Ralph. Tesco chief calls for laws to extend fight against obesity. *Times, Lond* 2013; December 26: 49.

42 Anonymous. Clear as coke: The world's biggest fizzy drinks maker is distorting the debate on sugar. *Ibid* 2015; October 9: 33.

43 Z Kmietowicz. Hunt is obstructing sugar inquiry, says MP. *Br med J* 2015; 351: 1.

44 C Smyth. Obesity report blocked by Hunt supports a sugar tax, MPs told. *Times, Lond* 2015; October 21: 4.

45 C Smyth. Boris close to backing tax on sugar. *Ibid* 2015; October 22: 16; Anonymous. Taxing Sugar: The arguments for a levy to help curb the epidemic of diabetes are too compelling for the government to ignore. *Ibid* 2016; January 6: 27.

46 Anonymous. Lansley's legacy: The coalition's hapless healthcare reforms are coming home to roost in red ink across the National Health Service. A blank cheque is not the answer. *Ibid* 2016; February 5: 29Anonymous. Don't Sugar the Pill: the government has delayed publishing an important report on obesity and public health. It must do so, and give serious consideration to a sugar tax. *Ibid* 2015; October 22: 31.

47 C Smyth, L Fisher. Pressure on Cameron to bring in sugar tax: health of our children at stake, NHS chief warns. *Ibid* 2015; October 23: 1, 8; D Lawson. Here's the bitter truth: a sugar tax will not make us thinner. *Ibid* 2015; October 25: 18; Op cit *see* note 25 (Griffiths, Shipman) above.

48 L Donaldson. A sugar tax is vital if we're to keep the NHS alive. *Times, Lond* 2016; January 5: 26; C Smyth. Pressure on PM as world health chief calls for sugar tax. *Ibid* January 26: 12; C Smyth, S Coates. Cameron hints at new sugar tax. *Ibid* 2016: January 8: 4.

49 C Smyth, S Coates. Sugar tax put back on table: cabinet swayed by evidence over obesity levels. *Ibid* 2016: January 7; 1, 10; C Smyth. Supermarkets will accept sugar tax on drinks. *Ibid* 2016; February 6: 16.

50 L Fisher. Olympic star joins call for tax on sugar. *Ibid* 2016: February 10: 6.

51 A Frean. Fizz returns for Coca-Cola as sales increase. *Ibid* 2016; February 10: 43.

52 L Fisher, N Badshah. Sugar tax is ruled out in obesity fight. *Ibid* 2016; February 13: 4.

53 F Elliott, S Coates, M Savage. Osborne sugars the pill: tax on soft drinks to raise £520m in childhood obesity battle: big business raided as chancellor predicts 'stormy waters' ahead. *Ibid* 2016; March 17: 1, 2; (*See also*: T Montgomerie. Nanny is right to limit our spoonfuls of sugar: the tax on sweet drinks makes sense for small-state Conservatives because it will reduce demand for public spending. *Ibid* 2016; March 17: 31; Anonymous Unsweetened medicine: caught between a global showdown and a Europe referendum, Osborne had little room for manoeuvre in the budget. What room he had he used well. *Ibid* 2016; March 17: 33; A Ralph. Soft drinks makers fall flat after sugar tax surprise. *Ibid* 2016; March 17: 53.)

54 C Smyth, A Ellson, D Walsh. Fizzy drink tax brings cheers but it's not to everyone's taste. *Ibid* 2016; March 17: 7.

55 T Fry. Fizzy drinks tax and the health of the nation. *Ibid* 2016; March 18: 32; G Coren. Never mind the sugar tax, we need a latte levy: don't be surprised that cups aren't being recycled. StarCosNero only care about peddling their fatty, revolting products. *Times 2, Lond* 2016; March 19: 20.

56 C Smyth. May rips up plans for junk-food crackdown: children condemned to obesity, experts warn: 'Sugar tax' on soft drinks survives. *Ibid* 2016; August 18: 1,2; T Rayment. May takes bite out of child obesity fight. *Sunday Times, Lond* 2016; October 30: 12. (*See also*: J Oliver. May's child obesity plan is all flab and no meat. *Times, Lond* 2016; October 30: 28. C Smyth. Make us sell healthy food, supermarkets implore May. *Ibid* 2016; August 9: 1, 2; D Sanderson. May 'abandoned battle against obesity because she is childless'. *Ibid*

2017; May 30: 17.)

57 K Gibbons. May 'ignoring' health cash crisis. *Ibid* November 5: 24. (*See also*: C Smyth. 'NHS heading for disaster' *Ibid* 2016; March 15: 14; C Smyth. Offer therapy to tackle obesity, NHS told. *Ibid* 2016: September 24: 13.)

58 J Russell. Children need our help in the war on weight: obesity in youth can blight the rest of our lives so ministers must do more than levy a sugar tax. *Ibid* 2016; November 17: 28.

59 C Smyth. Food giants reject lower sugar target. *Ibid* 2017; March 22: 1, 2; Anonymous. Sweet Nothings: if food manufacturers will not agree to cut sugar, the government must make them. *Ibid* 2017; March 22: 27; T Rycroft. Lower sugar target. *Ibid* 2017; March 23: 36.

60 C Smyth. Sweets must get smaller, health chiefs insist. *Ibid* 2017; March 30: 2; R Viner. The food industry needs to curb the nation's sweet tooth. *Ibid* 2017; March 30: 28.

61 C Smyth. Make excess sugar illegal to fight obesity, MPs urge. *Ibid* 2017; March 27: 4.

EPILOGUE

There can be no doubt, taking both historical facts and contemporary observations into account, that obesity is rapidly increasing throughout the world; this has already happened in the 'western world' (*see* Fig E-1) and is at present also taking place in 'third world' countries. Clearly, there is either an imbalance between input and output from a *calorie* perspective, and/or there has been a significant change in a common nutrient and/or its metabolites! A major problem is that it seems virtually impossible to obtain accurate figures (including calories consumed) or the extent of overeating, official estimates apparently bearing little resemblance to real amounts, which are invariably higher.[1] A lack of exercise is clearly also important in the equilibrium, there being no doubt that this is a major factor – especially in childhood. Not only are children walking less but, owing largely to the disposal of school playing-fields, they play significantly fewer sports demanding physical activity.

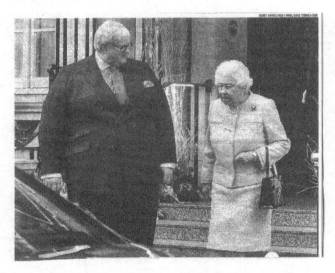

Fig E-1: *Times* photograph which, when originally published, was headed: 'A new level of Royal protection'! (V Low. *Times*, *Lond* 2016; December 8: 21 and 2017; December 13: 21.)

The outstanding alteration in everyday lifestyle however, is in eating habits, the most dramatic of which is a huge increase in consumption of both 'junk food' and 'sugary drinks'. There can be no doubt that *'refined-sugar'* consumption has steeply escalated during the last few decades. In the 1960s John Yudkin was aware that *'refined-sugar'* markedly raises blood triglyceride, cholesterol, and insulin concentrations; furthermore, it increases platelet stickiness and impairs glucose tolerance; however he did not pay attention to the separate contributions of individual *glucose* and *fructose* moieties of sucrose. It should be appreciated that his incrimination of *'refined-sugar'* as a *cause* of numerous medical problems was based on *epidemiological* data and an assertion that these all resulted from increased consumption of *total calories*. He did *not* question the fact that *fructose* (metabolised in a totally different manner to that of glucose (*see* Chapter 8) might be responsible; in fact, *fructose* itself could be *the* important 'toxic' factor! *Homo sapiens* from time immemorial has obtained a substantial quantity of his/her calories from glucose (or maltose); therefore, the 'abnormal' dietary component in the *twenty-first* century must be the astronomical quantity of *fructose* (the sole component apart from glucose) of sucrose (*ie, 'refined-sugar'*). The crucial link therefore surrounds the form in which *fructose* enters the portal system, *ie,* following absorption from the small intestine. A species variation is thought to exist, and it has been clear since the 1960s that most *fructose* in *H sapiens* reaches hepatocytes unchanged (*see* Chapter 8) but knowledge of this physiological fact has been largely ignored or disregarded! This book has clarified the nature of the moity of *'refined-sugar'* entering the portal circulation and hence presented to the hepatic cells.

Therefore, the major change to *human* lifestyle must be peaks of *fructose* entering the portal circulation following *'refined-sugar'* ingestion; *fructose* fails to stimulate insulin release (unlike glucose), and its metabolism incorporates both *triglyceride* and *uric acid* production. Furthermore, *fructose* does *not* affect *leptin* production (a hormone which signifies 'fullness'), and probably raises the concentration of *ghrelin* (a hormone which *induces* hunger).[2] Thus the colossal concentrations of *fructose,* liberated from *'refined-sugar'*, have an overall effect of 'persuading' an individual to eat more! This is therefore the major 'driving-force' behind being overweight or obese. In early primates, an enzyme handling large quantities of *fructose* which was perhaps 'switched off' for 'Darwinian' survival purposes, *ie,* to channel *fructose* to adipose tissue, might provide an *evolutionary* answer (*see* Chapter 4)[3] and also explains the reason for a high blood *uric acid* concentration and consequent epidemic of *gout reported* in recent years.

Present-day food supplies

A present-day problem is that there is a world *abundance* of food from a *calorie* perspective (including a significant excess of '*refined-sugar*'); unhealthy food and drink should of course ideally be made more expensive, which is certainly not the case at present. So much finance is involved, that governments are reluctant to intervene, largely for political reasons. Food wastage has as a result become commonplace! Our nearest approximation to a Malthusian scenario as a nation was during the *Second World War* – 1939–45 (days of food rationing); food had limited availability and there was little on which to feed this country's population. Sugar-containing foods and drinks were in very short supply. The British government formed a 'department' to identify optimal ways of food usage, (Lord [Frederick] Woolton [1883–1964]) became the British Food Minister (with willing input from medical experts) and identified correct constituents and vitamin content etc. Medical advice was then readily accepted, unlike the present situation! Never had the British population been in such good health; there was little obesity, while dentists became virtually unemployable – so unusual were dental caries.

Children are now so accustomed to purchasing food products from a local supermarket that they have no idea from whence they come (*eg,* some assume that potatoes grow on trees, and others that milk is obtained from bottles and *not* the cow). In some cultures, a knowledge of food and its medical sequelae goes side-by-side; this was probably the case in Britain in bygone generations, but over the centuries the two have become increasingly separated; the *Worshipful Society of Apothecaries of London*, for example, had its medieval origin in the Grocer's Company. During World War II (1939–45), the British population was encouraged to grow its *own* fruit and vegetables, often on an allotment, leading to far greater understanding of food-production.

Influence of government and the food industry on the obesity epidemic
The *food-industry* (in close collaboration with the British government), and with a major interest in shareholders dividends rather than individuals, has argued *against* the line of reasoning pursued in this book, and advertised and promoted both *sweet* foods and 'fizzy drinks'. Childhood obesity, they conclude, lies predominantly with other factors – headed by lack of exercise. Procrastination by government with a *tax* on '*refined-sugar*' allowed the obesity epidemic to escalate for far too long! Opponents of a '*refined-sugar*' tax in the *food industry* have sought to blame alternative factors for the pathogenesis of obesity. Writing in the *Journal of Sports Medicine*, a group of doctors maintained that there has been 'little change in population-wide physical activity ...' over the last thirty years, whereas during this time obesity has soared, and as a result it predicted future lawsuits criticising the food-industry for 'its rôle in (causing and encouraging) obesity'. Now, with a *new* Prime Minister (May), the future looks increasingly gloomy! Diminution of dietary '*refined-sugar*' is now a *voluntary* matter which is largely in the hands of the *food industry*!

In *summary*, reducing dietary *fructose* intake (together with increased exercise) is now *crucial*. However, to the medical scientist (myself included), knowledge of an underlying mechanism(s) behind being overweight or *obese* is essential, there now being little doubt that the *fructose* moiety of sucrose is largely responsible, and the fact that this monosaccharide is presented for metabolism *intact* following absorption, and this must be the essential component in the equation leading to obesity's *cause*.

In *conclusion*, four factors have contributed to the present *obesity pandemic*:

- Failure to realise that *fructose* is handled by the human body (and presented to the liver) totally differently from glucose, despite its calorific value being identical. A mechanism for handling these huge resultant concentrations of *fructose* does *not* exist in present-day *H sapiens*),
- Fraudulent publicity by an American 'scientist', which purportedly demonstrated that diets rich in fat and cholesterol were

pathogenic as far as human atherosclerosis was concerned. As a result, populations throughout the world substituted '*refined-sugar*' for fat as a major calorie source,

- Lack of *exercise* – resulting largely from overuse of the 'internet' and television. Children are now taken to school by car, instead of walking and taking public transport. Sale of school playing-fields has exacerbated the problem, and
- Dominance of the *food industry*, with opposition by the British government to reduction of '*refined-sugar*' in food and drinks. *Voluntary* reduction is simply *not* an acceptable policy.

With current realisation that *dietary* fat and cholesterol are *not* strictly relevant to the pathogenesis of obesity and atherosclerosis production, *normal* diets will perhaps resume, and consumption of '*refined-sugar*' will hopefully slowly decline. However, the problem with exercise-deficiency remains.

In any case, obesity is undoubtedly caused by an *environmental* factor, probably dietary (most likely '*refined-sugar*') to which the entire world population is exposed. The extent to which a genetic predisposition is involved is unclear.

References and notes

1 O Wright. Bad figures hid truth on how Britain is overeating. *Times, Lond* 2016; August 8: 13.
2 T O'Callaghan. Sickly sweet. *New Scientist* 2014; February 1: 35–40; S Luo, J R Monterosso, K Sarpelleh, K A Page. Differential effects of fructose versus glucose on brain and appetite responses to food cues and decisions for food rewards. *Proc Nat Sci USA* 2015; 112(26); 81: 36–41.
3 Chapter 8; J Leake. Obesity epidemic linked to chubby chimp gene. *Sunday Times, Lond* 2015; November 15: 27.
4 K Lay. Doctors accuse food companies of acting like Big Tobacco. *Times, Lond* 2015; April 23: 19.

ADDENDUM

Whilst in press, the journal *JAMA Internal Medicine* published, in 2017, criticism of research published in 1967 in the *New England Journal of Medicine* (before details of funding had been added). This research funded a 'campaign' launched by the sugar industry which was designed to indicate that saturated fat and *not* '*refined-sugar*' was a significant causative agent in coronary heart disease. Although fifty years old, this misleading contribution by the Sugar Research Foundation has a significant place in the position of '*refined-sugar*' in human nutrition and contains information indicating that '*refined-sugar*' and *not* saturated fat has significant side-effects.

INDEX

References to pictures are in **bold**; references to tables and figures are in *italics*

fizzy drinks
  amounts of sugar in 29, 41, 79,
  139, 139–140
  and caffeine 83
  and childhood obesity 28–29, 80,
  139–140, 184–186
  and sugar tax 192–217
  see also Coca-Cola; food industry
fluoride 110, 114
Flynn, Albert 190–191
Food and Drink Federation 187,
  203, 212
food industry
  advertising 11, 25, 189, 192, 200,
  201, 204, 213, 216
  and children 28–29, 154–155,
  184–185
  denial of role in obesity 42, 179,
  180–181, 187, 188, 190–191,
  193–198, 216, 227
  and developing healthier products
  178, 187, 193, 210–211, 212, 215,
  216, 217
  and independent experts 183–
  186, 190–191, 193–198
  labelling of products 84–85,
  138–139, 142, 179
  and sponsorship 193, 194, 195,
  196, 197, 198, 201
  and sugar profits 191
  sugar tax 192–217
  voluntary strategies 187, 208,
  212, 216, 217, 228
  see also Coca-Cola; fizzy drinks
food labelling 84–85, 138–139,
  142, 179
Food Standards Scotland 196
food supply 226
food waste xii, 85
Friedman, Jeffrey 105

fructose
  absorption products of 89–96,
  101
  clinical investigations of absorption of 89–101
  evolutionary hypothesis 38
  and gout 123
  and insulin 100
  metabolism of 95–101
  as trigger of obesity x–xi, xii, 37,
  96, 100–101, 225–226, 227
fruit and vegetables 46, 77–78, 81,
  82, 83, 84–85, 136–137, 138–139

G
gastric band 170, 171, 172
gastric bypass 106–107, 170–171,
  172, 175
gastric plication 170
general practitioner's role 17, 142,
  152–153, 191
genetic influences 39, 46–47
Gerard, John 61
ghrelin xi, xix, 100, 104–108
glucose 89, 90–95, 100
gout 38, 122–124, **122**, 137
government intervention 178–217
  2016 budget 211–212
  2017 budget 215–216
  and childhood obesity 199–203,
  213–214, 215–216
  and Coca Cola 195–198
  and food industry 179–188,
  190–199, 206, 210–217
  and salt consumption 180
  sugar tax 192–217
green tea 154
Greer, Germaine 3–4
gum disease 113